Thyroid Adrenal Weightloss Solutions!

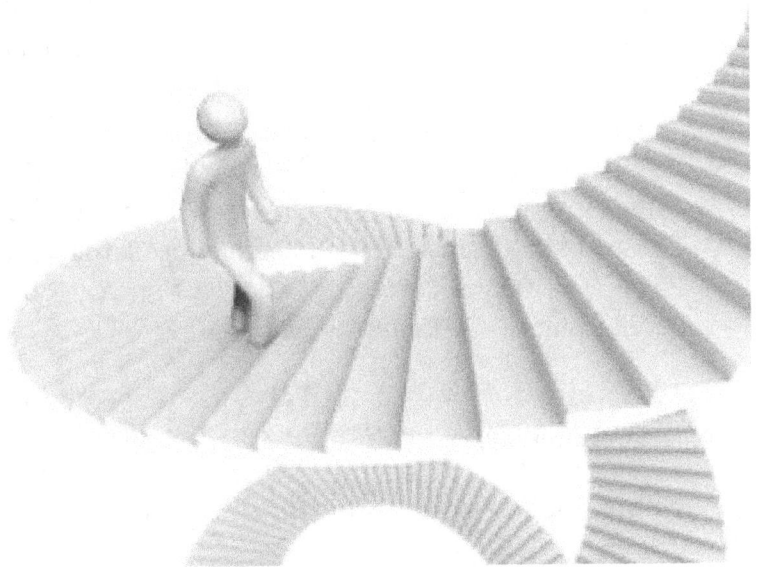

A 25 Step Guide

Attention: If you think you may have thyroid issues, if you feel something is holding you back from losing weight, if you feel tired, frazzled, maybe just a bit worn down, or you just want a guide to give you some natural, alternative, yet practical health tips and tricks leading to feeling super, this may be the guide you are looking for. Don't miss out – this information might change your life!

Other Books by ABC Wellness in the
"Simple Steps to Better Health" Series:

Calming Inflammation: The eBook "Autoimmune and Inflammation Solutions" gives you a Natural Recovery Protocol to Overcome Food Allergies, Gluten, GMOs, EMFs, Biofilms, Yeast or Candida Overgrowth. Only 99 cents!

Dental and Heart Care: The eBook, "Reversing Gum And Heart Disease" provides a Protocol to Lower hs-CRP, and Heal Inflammation Through a Paleo Diet, Dental Care, and Targeted Nutrients and Supplements. Only $2.99!

Thyroid and Adrenal Facts: The eBook "Thyroid Adrenal Secrets Revealed" teaches you what you the 10 top things you need to know before you see your doctor for thyroid or adrenal issues.

Analyze and Improve Your Health: The eBook "25 Step Healing Program" gives you simple steps to take to evaluate your health and improve it by correcting deficiencies.

Improve Your Health Safely: The eBook "Heal Your Whole Body Naturally" covers using bio identical hormones as well as a natural approach to staying well.

Lose Pounds Quickly by Overcoming Obstacles to Weightloss: The eBook "The ABC Wellness Weightloss Pyramid" covers 9 major obstacles or possible roadblocks that once removed will help you lose weight without dieting or exercise, though that is recommended to compound your gains.

Acid Reflux or GERD: The eBook "Acid Reflux Relief Now" allows you to stop heartburn or acid reflux in its tracks with natural remedies.

Anti-Aging Secrets: The eBook "Insider Bio Identical Hormone Secrets and More" covers the secrets you need to know to stay young and health with the use of natural hormones.

Longevity and Anti-Aging Advice: The eBook "How to Live to 100 – Top Dos and Don'ts" gives you the top 10 dos and don'ts you should follow if you want to reach and surpass the golden age of 100.

Thyroid, Adrenals and Weightloss: The eBook "Thyroid Adrenal Weightloss Solutions" covers the 25 steps in the "25 Step Healing Program" book, along with more information on losing pounds quickly.

Special note on Thyroid Adrenal Weightloss Solutions: This is a modified version of the "25 Step Healing Program" eBook, so please purchase this one if you want more information on losing weight as well as the thyroid, adrenal and testing information.

Please forgive us if any sites referenced in our eBooks are not operational when you visit them, and please try back later, as they may be under construction. Thank-you!

Thyroid Adrenal Weightloss Solutions:

A 25 Step Vital Guide
to Thyroid Testing, Thyroid Treatment,
Toxins to Avoid, Nutrients Needed,
Iodine and Thyroid Supplements
to take to Feel Better,
Lose Weight, Lose Fat,
and Have More
Energy!

Diane Culik, MD
Kyle Weed, editor

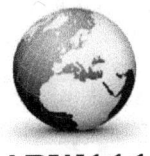

ABW111
ABW111 Publishing, Inc.
A Better World Company

Limits of Liability/Disclaimer of Warranty

Disclaimer: This information is for educational purposes only, and not meant to substitute for medical attention. If you have concerns with anything you want to try as a result of your learning here, please see your primary physician.

The authors and publishers of this book have used their best efforts in preparing this program. The author and publishers of this book make no representation or warranties with respect to the accuracy, applicability, fitness, or completeness of the contents of this program. They disclaim any warranties, express or implied, of merchantability or fitness for any particular purpose. The authors and publisher shall in no event be held liable for any loss or other damage, including but not limited to special, incidental, consequential, or other damages. The authors and publisher do not warrant performance, effectiveness, or applicability of any sites listed in this book. All links are for information purposes only and are not warranted for content, accuracy or any other implied or explicit purpose.

Table of Contents

CHAPTER 1: INTRODUCTION

WHAT IS THIS BOOK ABOUT?

This eBook provides a roadmap to thyroid adrenal health and health in general. It contains 25 immediate steps anyone can take to improve their thyroid adrenal health which may help them lose weight, have more energy, and just plain feel better than they do now. Please use the table of contents as a checklist and proceed through each item! And use your instincts or internal "hunches" as to what might be affecting you.

In other words, focus in on those areas you feel guided to – where you feel something might be going on and further investigation is merited. Your own wisdom can really help guide you to some meaningful answers many times, when an outsider would really have no idea without running multiple tests, and tests will often not reveal the truth completely. Think about your lifestyle, your habits, and your environment – could there be anything having an effect on you that you perhaps assumed was insignificant?

Be willing to experiment for a few days with a new way of doing things if you can – maybe what you discover will shed new light on what is going on. But one thing has become clearer and clearer over the years – many of us have been underactive physically, eating the Standard American Diet of refined and processed foods, and living with toxic exposures that really are not good for us – or our thyroid and adrenal glands.

(Helpful Tip: If you are reading this book, we believe you are probably beyond the basics as far as knowing what thyroid and adrenal glands are and how they work. However, as a refresher, and for some great information and explanations of how these glands work and what they do, please google "Thyroid" and/or "Adrenal" Glands, and check out some of the better sites with pictures like Web MD or Wikipedia.)

WHY WRITE A BOOK ABOUT THYROID AND ADRENALS?

Well, that's a good question. You see, right now there appears to be an epidemic of people walking around with thyroid issues and probably adrenal issues as well. It is estimated there are over 59 million people who may be experiencing some kind of thyroid problem, and most of them don't have a clue that this may be happening. Why? A couple of reasons seem apparent.

First, the soil is depleted of many minerals, including iodine, and iodine is critical for the thyroid to function. So the food you get in your grocery store in many cases does not contain sufficient nutrition to fuel the body properly. Recent tests in Michigan showed that over 95% of participants were low in iodine, so it's very possible that you are also.

14

Second, there are many toxins in the environment and in our food supply that affect us and our thyroid and adrenal glands and interfere with the functioning of these systems. It is important that you know what some of these toxins are so you can reduce or eliminate them from your life. We will cover more on both these issues later in this e-book, but suffice it to say that you are doing yourself a great favor by learning what the truth might be here.

Why is this important to you? What can you gain from knowing this? A lot - the benefits are myriad...

1. First, your health will be greatly improved by eliminating toxins and improving your diet and by ensuring you get adequate amounts of iodine and other critical nutrients. We will go over some of these items in this e-book.
2. Second, if you are overweight, the poor functioning of your thyroid may be the primary obstacle to why you cannot lose weight, and addressing this issue may mean major success.
3. Third, getting your thyroid and adrenals into proper shape will mean a less stressed out you. You will be able handles issues and challenges in your life a lot better when you have balanced your thyroid and adrenal glands.
4. Fourth, there is a lot of confusion about proper testing of thyroid and adrenals, and we will cover that also.

5. Fifth, following the advice we give may allow you to straighten out problem areas, and get into the best shape of your life through proper exercise and diet.

ABOUT THE AUTHORS - WHO ARE WE AND WHY SHOULD YOU LISTEN TO US?

This book is a collaboration between Diane Culik, MD, and Kyle Weed, independent health researcher. When two people work together, the end result of their efforts is often synergistic, and much more benefit is derived by the end consumer. What follows below is a write-up for each of us, and then a short explanation as to why we working together will benefit you as someone wishing to improve their health.

Dr. Diane Culik, MD, brings you natural health solutions, and is a top thyroid-adrenal doctor with over 30 years' experience! After graduating from the University of Michigan Medical School, Dr. Culik began practicing medicine a number of years ago, following the traditional path, learning the best that conventional medicine had to offer.

About 17 years ago, she switched to Holistic Medicine, and now blends the two approaches so you get the best of both worlds! She recently opened ABC Wellness, which stands for Alternative-Balanced-Comprehensive, in Sterling Heights, Michigan where she offers all patients "Simple Steps to Better Health." Her goal is to assist you in finding the path to a better way of life through the removal of obstacles to healing like environmental toxins and nutritional deficiencies and allowing the body to heal itself.

Kyle Weed is an independent health researcher, a writer, and communicator, with a "Vision" of reaching people through a variety of media and creating happiness, healing, and peace. He currently works with ABC Wellness to create eBooks, and DVD/Video Programs on Natural Health Topics such as anti-aging, cancer survival secrets, thyroid and adrenal care, weightloss, and more.

Kyle felt led to this experience through inner guidance after years of suffering through mercury toxicity caused in part by "silver" fillings, and after extensively researching the health field, reading through hundreds of health and medical books, websites and other literature. His goal is to bring Alternative Health Secrets, both ancient and new and unique Healing Modalities, Forgiveness and Mind Training Techniques and any other helpful healing information to public awareness.

How do the two of us working together offer a greater benefit to you, the reader, and user of possible life changing alternative health secrets?

By working together, the two of us fill in gaps each one of us working and writing independently may have missed. Dr. Culik provides the credibility of a trained medical doctor, can offer authoritative knowledge on many topics, and also the safety factor only a trained medical professional can offer, while still retaining a mind open to new and unusual alternative healing techniques. She will be the one providing the step by step instructions for this eBook based on her experience with patients, and her knowledge of thyroid and adrenal issues.

Kyle Weed, having undergone a lengthy health challenge and an equally lengthy period of studying health techniques and information can often definitively state in many cases what really worked to bring healing and comfort to himself and others undergoing similar experiences.

As I (Kyle Weed) am the one pulling the information together, and adding to it, I can state that I have personally read and studied tons of material from the leading alternative, natural doctors on the scene today, so both Dr. Culik and I will bring you the best of the best in alternative health care, including top secrets you can use right now! Please forgive us for any editing errors or formatting inconsistencies – we are still working to make this the best document it can be.

Disclaimer: Of course, we have to state that this information is for educational purposes only, and not meant to substitute for medical attention. If you have concerns with anything you want to try as a result of your learning here, please see your primary physician. Most things we mention are proven to be safe - foods, supplements, and testing methods you can try at home inexpensively, but please do err on the side of caution when trying anything. Start with small doses or trials and work up gradually if possible. This is especially the case when detoxifying the body. We provide more free information if you sign up at http://thyroid-adrenal-solutions.com, but we also recommend you work with a holistic practitioner who understands how to safely proceed.

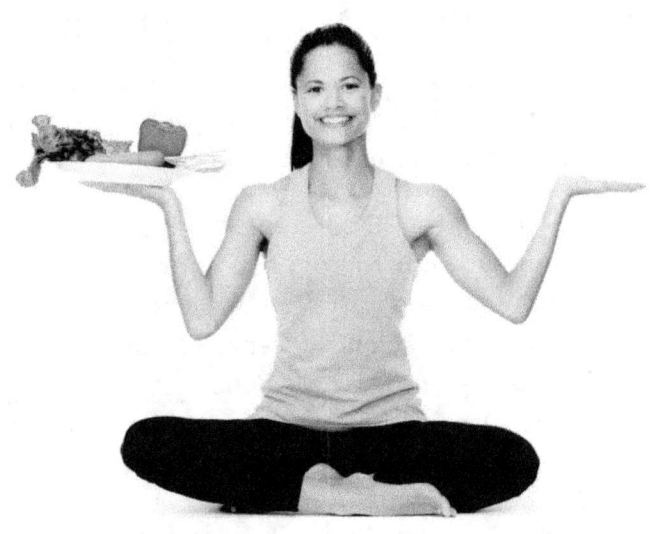

CHAPTER 2: STEPS 1 – 5, COMPLETE LAB TESTING FOR THYROID, COMPLETE PHYSICAL EXAM FOR THYROID, THYROID QUESTIONNAIRE, MORNING BODY TEMPERATURE TEST, AND FOOD ALLERGY TESTING.

Hi, I'm Diane Culik, and I would like to talk to you today about Thyroid Disease, and specifically "Is your thyroid disease being missed or mistreated?"

I want to go through 25 different things and steps or ways to improve your thyroid and adrenals that you need to know about to properly evaluate, treat, and improve your thyroid and adrenal glands. Are you afflicted with a thyroid issue? Follow steps 1-5 and find out for sure. If you are, you can start taking action to feel better immediately!

(Note: At the beginning of this manual there are a few questions that we had originally gathered some information from the internet in order to help answer the question. We have since removed that material as to not infringe on any copyrights. However, we will inform you to Google a certain subject, and you can read up on some great information and instructions to supplement what Dr. Culik has presented. Sorry for any inconvenience, but we strive to do things correctly.)

1. COMPLETE LAB TESTING FOR THE THYROID (FREE T3, FREE T4, TSH, TPO, ATG, REVERSE T3)

ONE, you need complete thyroid blood testing. A TSH test alone is not adequate to decide if you have thyroid disease. You really must know not only your free T3, free T4, TSH, your thyroid antibodies, which include TPO and ATG, but you have to know your Reverse T3 to see if you have inactive thyroid production. Anyone of those may be enough to indicate that you have thyroid disease. So if you don't have the whole panel, your physician isn't doing enough to evaluate your thyroid. (Google: Complete Thyroid Lab Testing)

2. COMPLETE PHYSICAL EXAM FOR THYROID CONDITIONS: SKIN, HAIR, NAILS, EYEBROWS, THYROID GLAND, PRETIBIAL EDEMA, REFLEXES

Number TWO, you need a complete exam for your thyroid. Thyroid Disease can be picked up on your blood work, but also many findings from your physical exam will suggest if you have thyroid problems.

You have to examine the skin for dryness, flakiness, and itching, and see if the hair is thinning. Nails can be pitted, and lateral brow thinning is a common problem; the thyroid gland itself can show nodularity or enlargement. Sometimes this is subtle, sometimes very severe. Pretibial edema can be obvious, or just some mild pitting or denting of the legs when you press on them with your thumb may be a finding. Also the reflexes of the lower extremities can be an indication of thyroid problems. (Google: Thyroid, Physical Exam)

3. REVIEW AND COMPLETE THYROID QUESTIONNAIRE OF SYMPTOMS: THIS WOULD BE HELPFUL TO TAKE TO AN OPEN MINDED DOCTOR

We have a complete thyroid questionnaire, number THREE, which may be a significant help in indicating if you have thyroid problems. You really need to go through this one by one, check off the items that seem relevant to you, and take this to an open minded physician, who can evaluate all your symptoms. A great place to start is to go to www.acam.org for Holistic Physicians. We have looked at your labs, your physical findings, and now your symptoms all by themselves may be a strong indicator of thyroid problems.

Thyroid Quiz and Symptom Evaluation (check any positives)

(____)   Sensitivity to cold or Hands and feet are usually cold

(____)   Morning temperatures are less than 97.8

(____)   Wear socks to bed often

(____)   Dry or scaly skin

(____)   Need to apply lotion and oils frequently

(____)   Often daily fatigue

(____)   Never seem to get enough sleep or naps for energy

(____)   Memory and concentration are decreased

(____)   Hair is thinning, course, dry, breaking off

(____)   Nails are thin, chip, peal or break

(____)   Lower legs are puffy, or indent with pressure

(____)   Hands and fingers are puffy

(____)   Carpel Tunnel symptoms

(____)   Outer third of eyebrows are thin or absent

(____)   Libido or sex drive has decreased or is low

(____)   Weight is difficult to lose or gain even when dieting

(____)   Bowels are sluggish or constipated or need to take laxatives

(____)   Autoimmune diseases like Rheumatoid, Lupus, and Vitiligo

(____)   Low B12 or Pernicious Anemia

(____)   Known or suspected food allergies or Celiac disease

(____)   Silver Amalgams now or in the past (Mercury fillings)

(____)   History of radiation therapy to neck or chest

(____)   Drinking now or prior, water with chlorine and/or fluoride

(____)   Eat moderate amounts of Soy milk, cheese, burgers, dressings, oil etc

(____)   Family History of any type of Thyroid Problems

(____)   Eat fish frequently esp. tuna, sushi, non-wild Salmon

(____) Moody, depressed, irritable, apathetic

4. MEASURE YOUR MORNING BODY TEMPERATURE (OK OVER 97.8). DOCUMENT FOR SEVERAL DAYS AND FOR WOMEN BEFORE OVULATION

Number FOUR, your body temperature is very important in evaluating if you have thyroid concerns, since the thyroid gland sets the metabolic rate. To check your thyroid, you can evaluate how your morning temperature is compared to normal, which should be 98.6, or maybe minus a degree. If it is less than 97.6, than you really have possible thyroid issues. Many people run 95 or 96 and their doctors tell them, "that's just the way you are, your temperature runs low." But usually there is a reason for it and most often it's because your thyroid isn't completely functioning. (Google: Basal Body Temperature Measurement)

5. FOOD ALLERGY TESTING IF ANY THYROID ANTIBODIES OR SYMPTOMS, ESPECIALLY IgG OR IgA ANTIBODIES FOR GLUTEN AND CASEIN

Number FIVE, is food allergy testing. This is something critical if there is any concern with thyroid disease and especially if you have elevated thyroid antibodies. Food allergies are so common today that probably everyone should have them done. And this has to be blood work with IGG or IGA blood tests. The skin test or IGE blood tests that an allergist or a pulmonary specialist might do are going to have

24

nothing to do with whether your food allergies are significant related to your thyroid. Those are going to be related to peanut allergy or asthma problems. But you have to specifically ask for and get IGG or IGA blood tests, especially for gluten, which is related to wheat; and casein, which a protein in dairy. (Google: Food Allergy Testing)

CHAPTER 3: STEPS 6 – 10, NUTRITIONAL CONSULTATION, HEAVY METAL TESTING, VITAMIN TESTING, SPECTRACELL TESTING AND THYROID TOXINS TO AVOID

6. NUTRITIONIST CONSULTATION IF FOOD ALLERGIES ARE DOCUMENTED TO ENSURE AVOIDANCE OF FOODS THAT ARE OFTEN A RISK

Number SIX, if you have any food allergy findings, anything positive, you really should see a nutritionist, and especially a holistic nutritionist to help you review what you are eating, what you can change, and how you can revise your diet. If there are several food allergies that are elevated, you may want to consider a complete blood panel of IGG blood testing, and several of the laboratories like Bio Tek are able to do that from even just a little finger stick of blood.

7. HEAVY METAL TESTING IF AMALGAMS, FISH INTAKE, OR OTHER EXPOSURES OR NEUROLOGIC SYMPTOMS SUCH AS TREMOR/ NUMB/ BRAIN FOG

Number SEVEN, heavy metal testing should definitely be done if you have any amalgams or silver fillings, if you eat or ever ate any significant amount of fish, certainly if you have exposures, just being near a coal factory that is coal burning. Also certainly be tested if you have any neurological symptoms, any tremor, any symptoms of Parkinson's, multiple sclerosis, any brain fog, chronic fatigue, fibromyalgia; all of these can be related to heavy metal toxicity.

8. Vitamin testing for Zinc, Selenium, B Vitamins, etc.

Number EIGHT, vitamin testing is very essential, and the things that are most related to thyroid problems are zinc levels, and especially red blood cell zinc level is important, your serum selenium is significant; those are both required for thyroid conversion in the cells to the active form (T4 to T3 conversion). And B vitamins are also essential, especially to measure B1, B6, and B12.

9. Spectracell Testing for Intracellular Nutrient Levels. Measure 33 including Vitamin C, K, E, Bs, Biotin, CoQ10, ALA, Selenium, Chromium, Calcium, Magnesium, Zinc, Copper, Glutathione, Inositol, Carnitine, Serine, Glutamine etc.

Number NINE, for more complete testing, there are labs such as Spectra-Cell that can do a very comprehensive analysis of intracellular nutrients, and they will measure 33 different vitamins, many that you can't get from a regular lab such as vitamin C, vitamin K, vitamin E, certainly all the B vitamins, but also Biotin, CoQ10, Alpha-Lipoic Acid, selenium, chromium, calcium, which is the only way to get an accurate level, not possible from traditional labs, magnesium, zinc, copper, glutathione, Carnitine, serine, glutamine, on and on. So this is a very helpful test, and everyone I have tested so far has one, and usually several deficiencies that are essential to correct for maximizing your health.

10. Avoid Soy, Fluoride, Bromine, Chlorine, PFOAs, Teflon

Number TEN, definitely avoid the toxic things that interfere with the thyroid and these absolutely are Soy, Fluoride, Bromine, Chlorine, PFOAs and Teflon. Soy, of course you know if you use Soy Milk or eat Soy Beans, but Soy is hidden in many foods, such as dressings and processed foods. Fluoride, of course you are probably going to have in your water, your shower, fluoride added toothpaste and mouthwash, so you want to get natural sources and filter your water. Bromine is very toxic. Bromo-Seltzer, brominated hot tubs, pretty much any processed flour now has bromine in it. And Chlorine is also in our tap water, great to kill off the bacteria, but damages the good bacteria in our gut and interferes with iodine. Teflon and PFOAs are also toxic and interfere with our thyroid. These are usually going to be in either plastic bottles or coated pans.

Thyroid Adrenal Weightloss Solutions

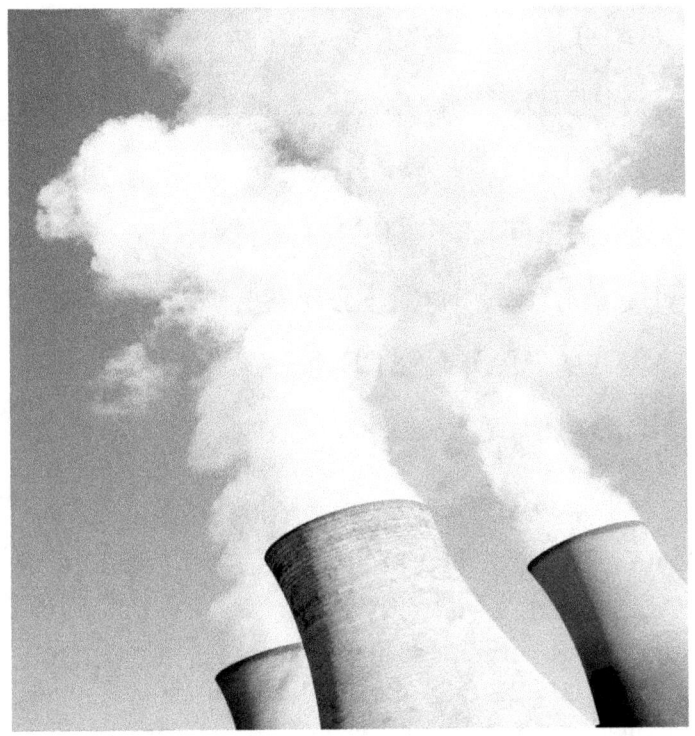

CHAPTER 4: STEPS 11 – 15, MORE THYROID TOXINS TO AVOID, ADEQUATE SLEEP, VITAL SUPPLEMENTS FOR THYROID AND ADRENALS INCLUDING VITAMIN C AND UNPROCESSED SEA SALT, LIVER DETOXIFICATION

11. AVOID MERCURY AMALGAMS, TOXIC VACCINATIONS (FLU SHOTS) AND FISH (OK PACIFIC WILD SALMON)

Continuing with more items to help your thyroid, Number ELEVEN is absolutely avoid any mercury amalgams, silver fillings have 50% mercury in them, also flu shots have, still, mercury in them, even though many vaccines have taken them out, and they put this in the vaccines they give adults as well as pregnant women and children. It's not good for your thyroid. Fish, basically limit to Wild Pacific Salmon, all other fish are going to have mercury in them and not worth the risk.

12. ADEQUATE SLEEP: USE MELATONIN (3-20 MG) OR HERBAL TEAS SUCH AS VALERIAN/ CHAMOMILE AS NEEDED OR GABA

Number TWELVE; you really need adequate sleep to support both your thyroid and adrenals. Very good for improving sleep is melatonin; you can start at 3 mg and you can double and triple the dose. It's very safe, and for people with immune deficiencies, or cancer, even 20 or 40 mg can be used. For other options, you can use herbal teas, chamomile, valerian, hops are very helpful, and GABA can be obtained in capsules, or now we even have the chewable GABA that not only helps sleep, but for anxiety and stress disorders.

13. ADEQUATE VITAMIN C 2-4,000MG /DAY IS REASONABLE, MORE FOR ADRENAL OR CHRONIC FATIGUE

Number THIRTEEN, vitamin C is good for every human being on the planet, and it's really critical for fatigue and especially for adrenal fatigue and adrenal burnout. Vitamin C is not made by human beings or other primates, also fruit bats and guinea pigs are not able to make vitamin C in their liver, we lost the ability, so we need to take in more vitamin C than just what is needed to prevent scurvy and die within a few months. We need it for our vascular system, our joints, our connective tissue, and absolutely for our adrenals – at least 2000 mg a day, is the preferred dose. It is available from Life Extension, from Pure Encapsulations, and you can get it in capsules, sometimes powdered, buffered form, and even chewable. It's excellent for kids to adults, any age. For adults at least 2000 mg, children, 1000 mg would be reasonable.

14. USE UNPROCESSED SEA SALT FOR ADRENALS (ONLY NON WHITE IS RIGHT—PINK, GREY OR BEIGE)

Next, number FOURTEEN, salt is very important for the body. Our bodies require salt, and you need to use unprocessed sea salt that is not white, that has all the good trace minerals in it. It may be Celtic or Himalayan Salt from deep deposits in the earth that have all the preserved natural minerals. If you have white salt, it is not the right salt, it has been made to look good, but they removed all the minerals. Sources (of unprocessed sea salt) are available from health food stores.

15. Detoxify the Liver with Herbs and Nutrients (Nutritionist or Naturopath) Milk Thistle, Alpha Lipoic Acid, etc.

Number FIFTEEN, it is very important to help support the liver, the adrenals, and the rest of the body to detoxify. And you can do that with nutrients, such as Chlorella, and Cilantro, or you can do it with many different herbs including milk thistle; also other nutrients such as alpha-Lipoic acid are very helpful. These are also available from Life Extension, and Pure Encapsulations.

Note – the below is pulled from an article we wrote earlier – you can sign up for these free articles at http://thyroid-adrenal-solutions.com. This also applies to Step 16 on Heavy Metal Detox that follows.

The suggestion is made to start with a trial first to see how you respond. There is a caveat with some nutrients such as chlorella and cilantro. Some practitioners believe these substances can stir mercury up and cause it to redistribute in the tissues, so proceed cautiously whenever using such items. Do this especially if you have a number of silver (mercury) amalgam fillings. It is recommended you have any silver fillings removed safely by a holistic dentist trained in proper removal, and replaced with safe materials. Ask your dentist to see the material safety data sheet for the filling material, and Google the ingredients for safety reasons.

Finally, whatever you finally choose to detox with, start with a very low dosage every few hours on a regular schedule and see how you do. There are support groups on the internet who will coach you in proper detoxification. Dr. Andy Cutler, a research scientist has written an excellent book on detoxing mercury from the body if you care to Google him as a resource – some consider him to be a premier authority on such issues. Detoxification products are available from Life Extension, and Pure Encapsulations.

CHAPTER 5: STEPS 16 – 20, HEAVY METAL DETOX, HERBS AND SUPPLEMENTS TO ELIMINATE YEAST, IODINE, VITAMIN D AND OTHER NEEDED VITAMINS AND MINERALS FOR THYROID AND ADRENALS

16. HEAVY METAL DETOX IF ELEVATED LEVELS (MAY USE ORAL DMSA, ZEOLITES, RECTAL EDTA SUPPOSITORIES, CHLORELLA, CILANTRO)

We are at number SIXTEEN, Heavy Metal Detox. If you have elevated levels of metals, THEY can be measured with urinary tests through several companies, including Metametrix. But we find if they are elevated you need to do something to pull them out, to loosen them up, and to get rid of them. And this will help free up a lot of heavy metals that interfere with thyroid production. Mercury pretty much binds the enzyme that converts T4 to active T3, and paralyzes that enzyme. So it will dramatically help your thyroid if you can eliminate heavy metals out of your system. Some of the options may include oral DMSA, Zeolites, which are used as pills, sprays, and drops, there are even rectal EDTA Suppositories and other herbal sources like Chlorella and Cilantro can be very helpful.

17. HERBAL, SUPPLEMENTS, MEDICATIONS AND NUTRITIONAL CONSULTATION TO ELIMINATE YEAST (LOW GLYCEMIC DIET, MANY HERBS ETC)

Number SEVENTEEN is yeast. It is fairly common in many conditions, especially in low thyroid. There are many ways to eliminate yeast from the body. There are prescription medications and there are herbal medications. Absolutely you have to follow a low glycemic diet, minimize sugar, pop, and very high glycemic carbohydrates such as white bread, white flour, and white rice. The herbs that are helpful include oregano oil and Olive Leaf, and oftentimes reviewing your whole diet with a nutritionist will help stabilize and eliminate yeast from your body, because otherwise it creates havoc and many symptoms - achiness, sore joints, brain fog, and definitely digestive problems with gas, bloat, constipation, and diarrhea.

18. IODINE AT 12.5 MG/DAY OR MORE FOR THYROID, BREAST, OVARIES, UTERUS AND PROSTATE (TYPICAL INTAKE HEALTHY JAPANESE)

Number EIGHTEEN is Iodine which is critical for everybody, but absolutely essential if you have thyroid problems. Our bodies don't get enough from the salt that we eat. The problem is that Iodine is only added to the white salt that has been processed and all the minerals have been removed. So what you want to do is use only the unprocessed, natural sea salt that is usually pink or gray, this will have no iodine, and what you really need to do is mimic what the Japanese people do, and take iodine pills or eat sea vegetables, or take kelp tablets and try to get your iodine intake up to 10 or 12000 mg per day, which is the average for the Japanese, who live longer on this planet than any other nationality. They also have the lowest rate of breast cancer in any developed nation for their women. Iodine is what your thyroid uses to create thyroid hormones, either 3 or 4 iodine molecules, and all the other chemicals we are exposed to like bromine, fluoride, chlorine interfere and block this iodine we are getting, so we need to make sure we are getting adequate amounts to keep the thyroid functioning.

19. VITAMIN D TO KEEP 25 HYDROXY-D LEVELS AT 50-80 (50% LESS BREAST CANCER WHEN VITAMIN D LEVELS OVER 52)

Number NINETEEN, Vitamin D is very important for health. It helps your thyroid; it lowers breast cancer risk, probably most cancer risks it lowers. It helps improve your immune system for flu, for infections, and it lowers the risk of diabetes, high blood pressure, and even multiple sclerosis. Your 25 Hydroxy vitamin D levels should be 50 to 80, and this is referenced per Dr. Hollick, who is a Vitamin D expert. Studies have shown that women have 50% less breast cancer when their vitamin D level is 52 or above. So it's very important to support your thyroid and your immune system by keeping your vitamin D levels adequate.

20. ADD VITAMINS AND MINERALS THAT ARE DEFICIENT (DOSES DEPEND ON LEVEL OF DEFICIENCY)

Number TWENTY is just to make sure that all the vitamins, minerals, nutrients that have been tested - that they are not deficient. Everything needs to work together in good working order, so your B Vitamins, your D, your Iodine, your Vitamin C, your amino acids, everything needs to be optimized for adequate and optimal   functioning.

Chapter 6: Steps 21 – 25, Adaptogenic Herbs, Saliva Testing for Adrenals, Food Allergy Panel, Probiotics and Nutrients for Gut Healing, and Natural Thyroid Hormone Therapy

21. ADAPTOGENIC HERBS AND NATURAL HORMONES WHEN NEEDED (ASHWAGANDA, GINSENG, RHODIOLA, PREGNENOLONE, DHEA, ETC)

Number TWENTY ONE is adaptogenic herbs and natural hormones, and these are very helpful to support the thyroid. You need to make sure your DHEA and Pregnenolone are optimized. For any adrenal concerns, multiple adaptogenic herbs including Ashwaganda, Ginseng, and Rhodiola, etc. will help for energy and vitality. When your adrenals are functioning well that will help your thyroid.

22. SALIVA TESTING FOR ADRENALS IF ANY FATIGUE, EXHAUSTION. TEST SALIVA 4 TIMES OVER 24 HOURS TO EVALUATE YOUR CYCLE

Number TWENTY TWO – Saliva Testing for Adrenals – if you have concerns and you're not sure, there are several companies including Diagnostics that will do a saliva test. Just do a little spit 4 times during the day and they can measure your DHEA and cortisol as it fluctuates through the daytime and evening. This is really much more accurate than one single blood test at one point in time. It will tell you if you are having adrenal fatigue or adrenal burnout, or high cortisol, maybe high stress; both of these may be detrimental to your thyroid function.

23. IF ANY FOOD ALLERGENS CONSIDER FULL FOOD ALLERGY PANEL FROM BioTek ETC WITH 96 REGULAR OR VEGETARIAN FOODS AND SPICES

Number TWENTY THREE is for food allergies. If you have one or two of the common food allergens such as gluten or casein you may want to consider a whole panel, because often with leaky gut there may be other foods that have caused problems and you have become allergic to them. Several companies, including Bio-Tek will test 96 different food allergens by IGG from just several drops of blood that you can even do at home. Use a finger stick for blood and put it on a little card, dry it, and send it off. It is a fabulous way to get a very complete analysis, with minimal cost and time.

24. PROBIOTICS AND NUTRIENTS FOR GUT HEALING INCLUDING GLUTAMINE, OMEGA 3S, ALOE, MSM, LICORICE, COLOSTRUM

Number TWENTY FOUR; there are several nutrients that are very important for your gut healing and for inflammation. If you have food allergies or if you have yeast then you probably have leaky gut. Healing nutrients may include glutamine, the omega 3's, or Krill Oil, Aloe, MSM, licorice, and colostrum.

Coconut oil is good for gut health, good for thyroid, good for improving your weight, and may even have some benefits for brain health. So coconut oil is another simple, easy thing that you can add as a nutrient into your body.

Probiotics are essential for everyone, but certainly if there is gut inflammation, if you have food allergies, or if you have yeast. Again, probiotics mean you are putting the good bacteria in to replace the bad bacteria and yeast, and function of the intestines is dramatically improved and it even helps for weight loss and for mood problems and mental health.

25. NATURAL THYROID HORMONE THERAPY AS INDICATED, PRESCRIBED BY A PHYSICIAN, FOR MEN AND FOR WOMEN

Last, number TWENTY FIVE, is utilizing natural thyroid hormone therapy like Armor or NatureThroid or West-Throid that your physician can order and can be obtained from a regular pharmacy; or compounded thyroid hormone from a compounding pharmacy. This can maximize the exact amount of T3 and T4 in your thyroid hormone pill by compounding it specifically for your needs.   This is essential to make sure you have both T3 and T4 levels that are adequate.

Please note that prescribing of natural thyroid hormone is the last step; there is a chance that by following all the previous steps in order that you may not need this medication. Perhaps adding in some natural foods or supplements and eliminating toxins will have you feeling top notch with no need for anything else. A natural remedy of the situation is always best, but many do find natural thyroid hormone to be helpful.

CHAPTER 7: TOP WEIGHTLOSS TIPS TO CONSIDER

OK, hopefully some of the steps you have taken above have removed the thyroid and/or adrenals as obstacles to weight loss, but we wanted to add a few more tips to help you get healthier and shed pounds. You may know some of these already, but it never hurts to go over them again. Let's list out some top tips:

1. Reduce your sugar intake to 25 grams or less per day. Yes, hard to do, but if you can, you will find losing weight a lot easier. Please don't underestimate the power of this step – this one point can let you have success losing weight! Many years ago, people consumed a fraction of the sugar they do today. If you are ever not feeling well, cut your sugar immediately. It can work miracles. Give this a try and keep track of your sugar intake and your body weight for the next 7 days and keep the grams as low as possible. You may be amazed at the result.

2. Get rid of the pop – if you must have it, drink it by itself as a treat away from meals. Not diet pop either, if you are going to give in, drink the regular kind, hopefully with real sugar and not high fructose corn syrup.

3. Avoid corn products of all kinds that have corn that has been genetically modified.

4. Eat only when you are hungry, and just enough to fill you up, skip the desserts.

5. Consider skipping meals occasionally, maybe even look into possibility of short term fasting. It has been proven in studies of mice that calorie restriction increases longevity, and it makes sense that humans can benefit from this strategy too. Think about it – it gives the organs a rest and the whole system a chance to purge toxins. The best and easiest way may be to have supper, begin your fast, and fast until the next day's dinnertime for a quick 24 hour fast. You might even do this once a week.

6. Try coconut oil – a tablespoon or so a day.

7. Concentrate on eating home grown or organic vegetables, with some lean protein.

8. Avoid refined, processed foods, eat as close to nature as possible.

9. Take a spoonful of quality flax oil and fish oil every day or two.

10. Resolve digestive issues with apple cider vinegar – just an ounce in a small glass, 3 or 4 ounces of water. A good choice is Bragg's Apple Cider Vinegar with the "Mother."

11. Here is one of the biggest secrets ever, and perhaps this should have been listed first. Instead of

worrying so much about losing weight, concentrate on increasing your strength and therefore your muscle mass as well. You can in a matter of a few months of real lifting transform your body in an amazing way. Of course, this is hard work, and you should clear with a doctor that you are ready for handling a heavy exercise schedule. This is not just for men anymore; many women have experienced the thrill of a new way of life through weightlifting. When you carry increase muscle mass around, your resting metabolic rate is raised, and you burn off excess weight easier. You also worry a lot less about diet, but by paying attention to both, you can change radically and quickly.

After saying all the above, we do have to make a statement to clarify things. We realize heavy lifting is not for everyone, just those who have real motivation for change. So, for most, plan to exercise moderately, even 30 minutes 3 days a week, and that will help boost metabolism; 5 or 6 days is better if you can handle it. Use weight lifting exercises as well as aerobics. Building muscle means you will burn more calories, and feel better too. You increase the oxygen getting into the cells, and you will also be able to fight off infections more rapidly too.

These are just a few tips to supplement other diet and or weightloss programs you may follow. Actually, the point is that if you go through all or even some of these steps, you may find yourself losing weight if you hit on one or more points or obstacles that need attention.

CHAPTER 8: CONCLUSION

In summary, we covered a number of topics including proper thyroid and adrenal testing, thyroid and adrenal toxins to avoid, as well as helpful supplements for thyroid and adrenals, critical nutrients, including iodine for thyroid and adrenal performance, and natural thyroid hormone therapy that, if needed, will help your thyroid's performance. The emphasis was on natural, alternative health therapies and solutions; solutions that would help you feel your best, lose weight, and have more energy, letting you live a less stressful life.

The benefits you gained from this e-book are hopefully many. If you proceeded through this book step-by-step, you will first know if your thyroid is afflicted, and then know how to treat it, what toxins to avoid, helpful thyroid and adrenal supplements to take, what level of iodine to take, and nutrients that can help you feel better, heal your gut, and boost your metabolism, including thyroid.

By buying certain food items, and being selective when purchasing food for your family, you can really improve the quality of what you eat. In addition, growing your own garden, and buying from local organic farmers who do not use pesticides is a great idea.

Another major benefit from application of what you learned is if your thyroid has been an obstacle to weight loss. Perhaps it may not be any longer with the

45

steps you have taken and you may shed unnecessary pounds. But whether you need to lose weight or not, having thyroid and adrenals that are in top notch condition will benefit you for life.

Thank you for joining us!

Diane Culik MD

ABC Wellness

Did You Like This Book?

Let everyone know by posting a review on Amazon. Just click here and it will take you to the reviews page; just scroll to the bottom.

CHAPTER 9: RESOURCE LIST

For your convenience, we have listed sources for supplements below. There is absolutely no obligation to buy, but we do appreciate it if you do. No matter where you make your purchase, please remember to buy only high quality items – your body deserves the best.

Here are sites you can go to for thyroid, adrenal, detoxification, hormonal and weight loss helpers that Dr. Culik approves of and are of high quality:

www.drculik.com (and go to the upper bar for NUTRITION)

- ThyroMedica Plus for enhancing thyroid function
  AdrenaMed for maximizing adrenal function
- T-100 includes freeze dried thyroid and adrenal gland plus minerals and herbals
- Weight loss, CLA Trim, MCT Oil to improve metabolic function, and Total Vegan Chocolate and Vanilla

Shakes that are not only gluten but dairy free so no whey or Soy
- Dual-Tox for maximizing liver cleansing for energy and weight loss

www.purecapspro.com/drculik. For vitamins and minerals and natural mood therapies

www.mydoterra.com/abcwellness. For essential oils for mood, hormonal support, for weight loss, detoxing, yeast infections and other infections including Lyme disease

Http://dianeculik.isagenix.com. For complete protein drinks either whey or nondairy, IsaCleanse for detox and weight loss...Ionix supreme for adaptogenic support of thyroid and adrenals...e+. Energy drink for natural boost of energy and metabolism

www.purerxo.com/ABCwellness

www.dssorders.com/ABCWellness
HCPC374WELCOME, DC374, $100

Shop anytime online
Website:
Registration Code:
☑ Order by Phone toll free: **877-846-7122**, 8:00-6:00 CST
☑ Enroll in Auto Ship for automatic deliveries — FREE shipping and 5% off.
☑ Rewards: Purchases earn points for future savings

Thyroid Adrenal Weightloss Solutions

- ☑ Free shipping on orders over
- ☑ Coupon: Save 10% on your first order →

CHAPTER 10: CHECK OUT THESE SPECIAL OFFERS!

We have found some other programs you may be interested in. The ones listed next are now available – just click to see the presentations on each topic on the following page. There is no obligation to buy, but these may give you the results you seek:

- The Beyond Diet Program: All Natural Diet, Click to view presentation
- Total Wellness Cleanse: Natural Food Based Cleanse!
- Coconut Oil: Boost your Metabolism and Get a Free Book on use with your Purchase!
- Sleep Program: Learn how to get better sleep!
- Bodylastics: Inexpensive, Excellent Exercise Program with Bands!
- Candida: Stop yeast infections now!
- Hypothyroidism Exercise Revolution: Better way to exercise if you are hypothyroid

To supplement the chapters above, we have included some questions and answers from a recent session at ABC Wellness. We hope you find the answers informative and helpful. Some of the information you may know already, but look them over and see if you can benefit.

BONUS: QUESTION AND ANSWER SESSION NUMBER ONE

1) Will this information be made available to us?
2) Have you written a book?
3) Do your handouts come with the recommended dosages of the supplements?
4) I am curious, artificial sweeteners, and diet pop, I have heard a lot about aspartame, can you comment on this?
5) What about Stevia?
6) I have a question, on one of your slides; you say that vaccinations are causing a problem. What is your take on that?
7) My main question was about vaccinations for babies and children as there has been a lot a controversy lately – what is your take on this?
8) I have a daughter with autism, and they gave her a last vaccine when she was two years old. At first I didn't care much about these stories, and I did not believe it. But she turned two years old and she got the vaccine, and she regressed. My second daughter, I did not do any vaccinations until she was a little older, not when she was a baby, but when she was older, in her preteens and teens, but I was very conflicted about it, any thoughts on this?
9) Why do all these hospitals require vaccinations?

Start Answers:

Will this information be made available to us?

We are working now to prepare it and it probably will be in an e-book form, maybe a video and it may be posted on our websites, you can check it www.drculik.com and http://www.abcwellnessnews.com. But you can also go to Amazon.com and type Dr. Culik and you will find my books that way.

Have you written a book?

We have posted a few e-books on Amazon.com so far, and we have some video presentations made of some of our talks, one on thyroid, one on bio identical hormones, one on acid reflux disease, you can Google, Amazon, and Dr. Culik and find my books that way, or go to Amazon Kindle Books and type Dr. Culik.

Do your handouts come with the recommended dosages of the supplements?

The e-books and the videos will have the dosages as I recommended them, you can check again on Amazon.com.

I am curious, artificial sweeteners, and diet pop, I have heard a lot about aspartame, can you comment on this?

Well, NutraSweet and Aspartame, they change the name so people don't recognize it, and it causes neurological damage, when they first tested it caused holes in the rat's brains, it never should've been on the market –

there was a big controversy. So Searle made it and then hired a couple of the FDA people who were investigating them, hired them over to work at Searle, bought them out, and the FDA dropped the case.

What about Stevia?

Stevia is natural, and xylitol's okay. No NutraSweet or Splenda.

I have a question, on one of your slides; you say that vaccinations are causing a problem. What is your take on that?

When I started out, I thought the best thing I was doing for patients and I wrote an article about it, was getting them to have flu shots. I no longer recommend flu shots, if patients want them, I will send them somewhere. But I haven't gotten flu shots in years. Flu shots still even today have mercury in them, although they have taken steps to pull the thimerosol out, it is still in some of them.

My main question was about vaccinations for babies and children as there has been a lot a controversy lately – what is your take on this?

Many of the children I see, and I don't see that many kids, I mainly see people middle age and older, usually the kids I see, usually their parents don't want vaccinations for them, and they are looking for a doctor who will support them in that. My receptionist has never had a vaccination on her three kids and even before she started with me. I am recommending that she probably start a few now. But I've seen a lot of healthy kids who have not had vaccinations and I definitely don't think you need to get the hepatitis B shot at birth, because it's for people who are going to be sexually active or shooting up drugs. It was going to be for teenagers, and they couldn't get them to do it. So the schedule, the amount of vaccinations, I talked to many, many families at the autism conference I went to and almost to a person they said at age 13 months or 18 months their kid stop talking after their vaccines, this came out in story after story after story. They absolutely believe it, that it is the vaccinations.

I have a daughter with autism, and they gave her a last vaccine when she was two years old. At first I didn't care much about these stories, and I did not believe it. But she turned two years old and she got the vaccine, and she regressed. My second daughter, I did not do any vaccinations until she was a little older, not when she was a baby, but when she was older, in her preteens and teens, but I was very conflicted about it, any thoughts on this?

There's a website called www.cdautism.org, for chlorine dioxide, and there is a woman in Mexico, I think she's American, but she's in Mexico who is curing kids using chlorine dioxide. Using it orally, and as enemas plus nutrients, and absolutely no wheat, no dairy, but using probiotics, and she is normalizing kids, absolutely, back to normal.

Why do all these hospitals require vaccinations? I have written a lot of letters trying to get people out of it, but it is such an accepted practice, you do what you can.

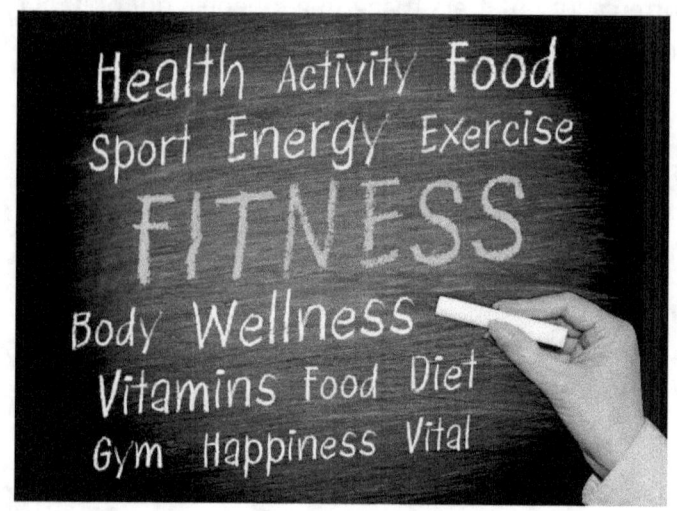

Bonus - Question and Answer Session Number Two:

1) What is the Paleo diet?
2) There's been a lot of in the research about Carnitine, I hear that it helps for energy and weight loss, but lately it seems the bad news about Carnitine, you heard anything?
3) So you went through a lot of information here – how does one get all this information if we were not able to take all the notes?
4) What do you think about Spirulina? Is a good for you?
5) And look at the fluoride; they put it in toothpaste – what you think of that?
6) How do you get good water?

What is the Paleo diet?

Basically they are looking at what did our ancestors eat, not our grandparents, but what the cavemen ate, what was natural. They are addressing the question of should we all be vegetarians, or should we all eat meat, or both? What kind of vegetables and meat?

Their theory is that our ancestors ate a mix of proteins and vegetables that they would just pull and harvest. So they were not doing grains, they were not farmers out farming wheat and corn or rice or something. So they ate meat, and they obviously ate a lot of vegetables, and they basically had all kinds of combinations of those things.

The more you can do, as most people think, of the wild, the organic, the grass fed kinds of proteins, (although sometimes they're very high in protein), and less of the more complex grains and vegetables the better. So no potatoes, no beans either. Basically, they are doing the asparagus and a slab of meat, that kind of thing.

There's been a lot of in the research about Carnitine, I hear that it helps for energy and weight loss, but lately it seems there has been bad news about Carnitine, have you heard anything?

Yes, as I just said some people are just going to eat their Carnitine and their red meat – I just saw an email on that. But obviously there's a difference of opinion there. Listen to the experts – I don't know the complete answer there – it might be good to do some research on the topic.

So you went through a lot of information here – how does one get all this information if we were not able to take all the notes?

Well, I have a handout that you get after you fill out your evaluation form. This handout has a summary of the resources, the websites, the books, the magazines, the types of test, the things to look for, and if you put your email on there when the information is pulled together, I think we're going to be sending out an email summary, so you can just go on that document online and click links, so that will make it easier and we will probably posting it on my website at www.drculik.com or at www.abcwellnessnews.com.

What do you think about Spirulina? Is it good for you?

I think so; I think it's is very good for health, and has lots nutrients, lots of vitamins, I don't specifically mention it here, but it is supposedly very packed with lots of good nutrients, so it is a good thing to add as a supplement or throw in a protein shake. A lot of the greens powders that I've used will have Spirulina as one of the ingredients in them. And you can get a lot of things in bars and shakes - whatever kind of form it comes in.

About fluoride; they put it in toothpaste – what you think of that?

Well, as much as we can minimize putting more fluoride in our systems we should, as well as maximizing the iodine to flush it out, but just as much we should also minimize putting more mercury and bromine in our bodies; we need to do the best we can at this.

How do you get good water?

Well, lots of people have different answers to that, I have a filter that I use here, and I have one at home. I used Nikken filters, but there are different water filters out there like Kangen Water Filters; there are a lot of companies that are probably pretty good, and I think that most of us should start with some kind of way to filter water.

If you do reverse osmosis, then make sure you're getting your minerals back in, whether through sea salts or through supplements; that's the way some people do it, you are also concerned about how is the pH going to be - not only is the water pure, but is the pH okay, can you add something in to balance the pH? Water is so good for us, yet you go to most stores, and it's all in plastic water bottles and it's been sitting out in the heat on a truck, filling it with more toxic chemicals, so it may be no better than tap water.

(Note: At this point a few other people brought up some things they learned about water that was interesting so we present it here. Research "Dr. Blaylock and distilled water," but for our purposes, we recommend pure water through filtering or reverse osmosis, and supplementing vitamins and minerals if needed.)

Speaker #1: And distilled water is not water you really want to drink because it is really mineral deficient, so you're actually going to find people who got sick from drinking distilled water. When it goes through the body, they talk about that water has a memory, and it binds to the minerals and leaches those minerals back out of the body, so distilled is definitely not a good choice if you're buying bottled water. You're better off buying spring water.

Speaker #2: Well do you remember Dr. Blaylock? He likes distilled water – it is in his newsletter. Well, maybe he put something back in the water too.

Dr. Culik: And of course he takes all kinds of minerals and supplements and stuff – maybe that's how he adjusts for that. And if you are not where you can get anything else, I guess that's an option, but if you can use some kind of good filter for your water, it is probably better.

(So there seems to be some controversy there. But at least consider using a filter, that's probably a good option here.)

BONUS: HEAVY METAL TOXICITIES, CHEMICALS AND BPA/PHTHALATES

(Note: This chapter is directly from our eBook called "The ABC Wellness Weightloss Pyramid.)

Chemicals and other toxins like heavy metals and BPA/Phthalates compose the last obstacle we will cover in our Weightloss Pyramid model. Again, so often people talk about chemical toxicities, heavy metals, pesticides, and phthalates as causing a problem or difficulty for those trying to lose weight.

TOXICITIES - SYMPTOMS

1) Fatigue and Chronic Fatigue Syndrome
2) Muscles Aches and Fibromyalgia
3) Difficult Weight Loss
4) Brain Fog
5) Fluid Retention
6) Low Thyroid
7) Numbness
8) Tremors, Restless Legs and Parkinson's

It has been reported that airline stewardesses, because of the chemicals sprayed in the cabins, the fire retardants, have a lot of chemical toxicities. But for the rest of us, there are certainly others who have exposures that may be harmful too. This includes people that might work in salons; persons doing hair and nails with toxic solutions, painters, and more. Definitely anyone who comes in with chronic fatigue and fibromyalgia, difficult weight loss, brain fog, fluid retention, low thyroid, and other issues like tremors, restless legs, and Parkinson's may have some contamination issues going on.

TOXICITIES - HISTORY

1) Prior or current Silver/Mercury amalgams
2) Prior or current Fish Intake esp. Tuna or Local
3) Prior or current Plastic Water Bottles
4) Prior or current Pesticides/Herbicides
5) Prior or current Tap water with Fluoride/Chlorine
6) Prior or current Bromine in Hot Tubs/Bromo-seltzer/Mountain Dew, Brominated (all) Flour
7) Prior or current flight in planes --- High Fire Retardant Sprays especially Pilots and Stewardesses

To address history of exposure, it may be silver fillings, fish intake, plastic water bottles, or pesticides. And you'd be amazed by how many people are spraying pesticides and chemicals in and around their house. Tap water can be toxic due to fluoride and chlorine, there is bromine in hot tubs and in airplanes the fire retardants may pose a problem. Try to be aware of what might be a toxin you need to avoid, and be careful when you have to use something potentially harmful.

TOXICITIES – EVALUATIONS

How do we evaluate people for toxicity? There are tests that can be done.

1) Urine Testing can be accurately done for heavy metals as long as a chelating chemical is used
2) Urine morning test for Phthalates and BPA
3) Testing is available for Pesticides

4) Testing can be done for other toxins

People can be urine tested with chelation to look for heavy metals, and there is a urine morning test for phthalates and BPA, and other tests exist for pesticides and other toxins. So, lots of companies have different specific tests and you should be able to find out more by researching the internet.

TOXICITIES – TREATMENTS

Here is a treatment list for exposure to toxic chemicals:

1) Identification leads to specific therapy for toxins....and helps avoid future exposures
2) Oral detoxification is possible with Zeolites, DMSA, Chlorella, Cilantro, EDTA-for metals
3) Detox pathways are improved with Methyl Folate, pure water, alkalinity
4) N-Acetyl Cysteine and Glutathione

As to treatment of toxicity, sometimes people say they just want to treat themselves and they can do oral detoxification with Zeolites, DMSA, Chlorella, Cilantro, and EDTA for metals, but whatever you do, please proceed cautiously and it is really recommended you consult with an experienced Health Practitioner who has dealt with numerous patients with the condition you suspect so you get an idea of how the detoxification process should normally proceed. This is especially helpful if you are not feeling well and do not know what to expect or how your body will react. Cleaning out the liver helps the body to detoxify and move the toxins out of the body and probiotics will help keep the bowels moving. But it is important to do it right, so expert help is always a great idea.

To continue with treatment of toxic chemicals, it is important to detox the liver phase 1 and 2 metabolism pathways. Here's what we recommend at ABC Wellness:

1) Dual-Tox from Numedica—includes Artichoke, ALA, NAC, MSM, Ellagic acid, Silymarin, Cal D Glucarate
2) Paleo Cleanse Shakes_from DFH with similar ingredients. Add to protein shakes or alone
3) ABC Wellness also uses Herbal Teas for Liver Detox and has a naturopath available for consultation

Some of the specific toxic chemical treatments I use include Dual-Tox from Numedica, which has many great ingredients in it. And there is a Paleo Cleanse Shake available that is a powder you can put in a protein shake or use alone - it is from Designs for Health (DFH) and has similar ingredients as Dual-Tox. Also, here at ABC Wellness, we have a Naturopath who has herbal teas for liver detox that she uses, so that is another option.

Here's more on treatment for chemical toxicities:

1) Amino acids, minerals, vitamins and omega 3s or Krill oil help--Glycine detoxes Phthalates and BPA
2) Paleo Cleanse from DFH: Powd-vit, min-Chrom/Vanadium, Aminos, Ca-D Glu, Taurine,

Silymarin,MSM, Inositol, Quercetin, Green Tea, NAC, Choline, Methionine, Dandelion, Glutathione
3) Good bowel function helps prevent reabsorption of toxins. Adequate magnesium, fiber and probiotics are part of the plan.
4) Cleanse drinks like herbal "<u>Isa-Cleanse</u>" from Isagenix removes toxins from fat.... to mobilize fat and fluids and maintain weight loss.

Again, when taking these supplements, make sure you're getting plenty of good amino acids, and Omega 3's. Paleo Cleanse has many helpful nutrients like Silymarin, green tea, and glutathione as well as many more. Also, make sure you are getting adequate amounts of magnesium, fiber and probiotics as this will help bowel function. Finally, ISA Cleanse is another product I've used over the years; it is from Isagenix and it helps clean the toxins out of the fat, and it helps to mobilize fats and fluids and to maintain weight loss.

What we covered should give you a good start on treating toxicities, but there may be other methods and supplements recommended by your own holistic practitioner. Whatever you do, proceed cautiously and safely, and research as much as you can about whatever methods you choose to use. If you experience discomfort when detoxing or cleansing, consult an expert you can trust on if it is OK to proceed.

If you liked this chapter and would like to learn more on the 9 obstacles, please use link below.

Lose Pounds Quickly by Overcoming Obstacles to Weightloss: **The eBook "<u>The ABC Wellness Weightloss Pyramid</u>" is live at Amazon and is available for purchase.**

BONUS – SMOOTHIES FOR WEIGHT LOSS AND SUPERIOR HEALTH

Smoothies are an excellent way to get vital nutrients in your daily diet, and if used with the proper ingredients and amounts, to lose pounds as well! Pick your favorite ingredients, and use the guidelines below to start. Modify recipes as you see fit, but try to do a bit of research on what items will best benefit you.

By concentrating on the elements you tend to lack in your daily diet, a daily smoothie may just be the answer you need to bring you up to maximum health and weightloss if desired. So, take the time to think about what might be the most beneficial smoothie you can make, and choose those ingredients to try. You can rotate with different recipes for variety as well in case you feel it's always the same old thing, and you want a new kind of taste.

Here is some basic guidance when preparing your smoothies.

Things to avoid:

Avoid NutraSweet and Splenda
Avoid Plastic water bottles for water source or drinking water

Avoid sugar, Agave and Honey if you are looking for weight loss.

Avoid Bananas--high glycemic and almost everyone I test is allergic and making antibodies to bananas

Avoid Dairy unless you have been tested for Casein and Whey and make no IgG Antibodies...a majority of patients I test are reactive to dairy and inflammation aggravates weight gain

Equipment Needed:

Use a Vitamix or Bullet or other powerful blender

Basic Items to Include:

Use a source of filtered water if available such as Nikken

Sweeteners - OK to use Stevia, Xylitol and/or B-Sweet from Boresha

Protein powder: Recommend Vegan from Numedica, Hemp powder, or Pea or Paleo from Designs for Health. The Paleo powder is sourced from Swedish cattle which are grass fed without pesticides and hormones. It is available in Vanilla or Chocolate.

Detoxification Nutrients You Can Add:

Paleo Cleanse Powder from Designs for Health

Raw sprouts, Ground flax seeds, Chia seeds

Radiant Greens powders from Tony O'Donnel, www.radiantgreens.com or Paleo Greens from Designs for Health, or Numedica Greens in Chocolate or Fruits and Greens in Strawberry-Kiwi flavors

Fruit Powders from Tony O'Donnel, or Designs for Health, or Numedica - also great options are

Pomegranate powder, Blueberry powder, Acai powder, available from Amazon and others
Raw organic greens such as Kale and Spinach
Fresh or Frozen organic berries such as blueberry and raspberry
Fresh organic apples 1/2 to 1 added with skin.

Thickeners:

You can thicken with coconut milk, coconut half and half, coconut yogurt, coconut kefir. Use plain preferably without sweeteners. Before using almond or rice milk make sure you have IgG allergy testing since many people are allergic to these.
Oils such as 2 TBSP Coconut, or Flax Oil, or half an avocado
Bananas if not looking for weight loss.

More Flavor and Detoxification – try Essential Oils:

For detoxification and flavor you can add 1-2 drops of essential oils such as Lemon, Orange, Grapefruit, Lime from doTERRA which are safe and effective internally to help break down fat cells
Natural Oils such as Lemon and combinations like On Guard are fabulous for safe and very effective natural cleaning products to add to water and vinegar and avoid toxic chemical sprays and cleaners that can increase weight.
SLIM AND SASSY is an oil combination specifically meant to be added to water to help with weight loss by controlling appetite and dissolving fat cells.

Smoothie Recipes for Energy and Weight Loss

Lemon/Raspberry Smoothie

1 scoop Vanilla Pure Paleo Powder from Designs for Health
12 oz. pure water
1/2 cups raspberries fresh or frozen
2 drops Lemon Oil from doTERRA
1 Tablespoon Flax Oil
1 Tablespoon Ground Flax seed
1 scoop Paleo Cleanse powder from Designs for Health
1 scoop Paleo Greens from Designs for Health

Chocolate/Orange Smoothie

1 scoop Chocolate Pure Paleo Powder from DFH
1 scoop Paleo Cleanse Powder from DFH
1 scoop Radiant Greens from Tony O'Donnell
8 oz. coconut milk
1 Tbsp. Flax Oil
1 Tbsp. soaked Chia seeds
2 drops Wild Orange Essential Oil from doTERRA
4 oz. pure water

Fresh Lime Smoothie

1 scoop Numedica Vegan Vanilla Powder
8 oz. Almond Milk
1 scoop Numedica Power Greens
4 oz. pure water
1 Tbsp. Ground Flax Seed
1 Tbsp. MCT Oil
3 drops Lime Essential Oil from doTERRA

Optional Additions

For Leaky Gut: Glutamine Powder 1/2 - 1 tsp. at 2-4000 mg from Life Extension

For Joint Health: MSM Powder 1/2 tsp.

For Immunity: Vitamin C Powder-Buffered 2-4000mg from Life Extension

For Immunity and Sugar: Bitter Melon powder 1 tsp.

For constipation, headaches, muscles cramps: Magnesium chelate powder available from Prothera etc

For Detox and Fluid Retention: Add Cleanse for Life Powder from Isagenix

Extra Nutrients: Organic Raw Spinach, Kale, Apple, Berries

Note: Many people are allergic to Bananas and also Strawberry is a frequent allergen so I usually avoid them

References:

For **doTERRA Oils**, go to:
http://www.mydoterra.com/abcwellness/

For **Numedica products**, go to: www.drculik.com and look for NUTRITION across the top - you can search for the following terms on the site to see helpful, related products: Adrenal Support, Thyroid Support, Detoxification, Gluten Sensitivity and Metabolic Management for supplement support.

For **Designs for Health**, as well as **Prothera Probiotics**, B12/Folate and more, go to: www.dssorders.com/abcwellness and use access code "dc374" to order - you can search PALEO for shakes and greens powders etc.

For **Pure Encapsulations** supplements and vitamins go to: www.purecapspro.com/drculik - go to ALL DEPARTMENTS and scroll to WEIGHT LOSS SUPPORTS (Options include: Chromium, Cinnamon, CLA, Pure Clear Powder, Pure Lean Nutrients, Pure Green Coffee Packets and more)

Thank-you again for joining us and good luck on your journey to a healthier, you!

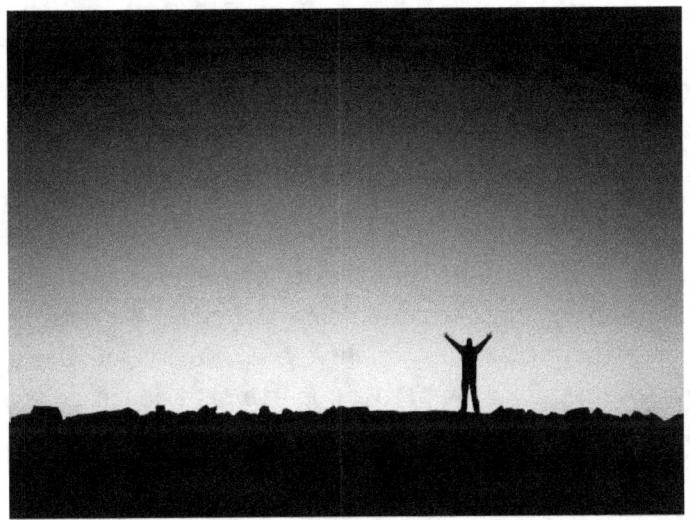

BONUS: ESSENTIAL OILS FOR HEALTH AND LONGEVITY

How would you like to upgrade your healthcare today naturally, without expensive medications and doctor's visits, saving you time, money and decreasing stress and aggravation? Is this even possible? Could it really be true? The answer is now a resounding yes, and it comes through the use of Essential Oils. Essential Oils are a hot topic these days, and becoming more popular as people realize the benefit of using them to stay healthy.

They come from the heart of plants and are considered "Nature's Medicine Cabinet". But please remember that the quality and purity of these Essential Oils are vital to a positive experience, so try to find ones of high quality. Your body deserves the best, so choose wisely.

The ones that I use and represent are called doTerra. Only doTerra offers Certified Pure Therapeutic Grade (CPTG) Essential Oils and Supplements. They are Certified Pure Pharmaceutical Grade (CPTG) and many of them can be inhaled as vapors or applied topically on the body, especially on the feet. They also can be taken internally by mixing with water or putting them into capsules. Here is more information on how I personally use these essential oils, but certainly, you may find your own favorite ways to apply them.

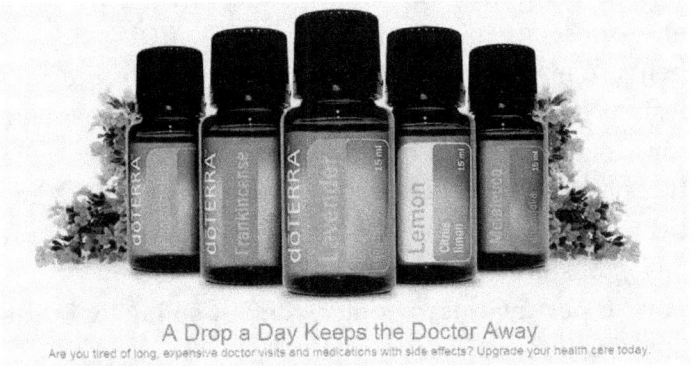

A Drop a Day Keeps the Doctor Away
Are you tired of long, expensive doctor visits and medications with side effects? Upgrade your health care today.

OnGuard is one of my favorites and is a combination of Wild Orange, Clove, Cinnamon, Eucalyptus and Rosemary. I carry a small bottle of "beadlets" in my purse and pop 2 or 3 in my mouth to freshen breath or at the first sign of any throat irritation. The outer cover dissolves and gives a fresh blast of cleansing oils. I also use the pure oil to put drops into a capsule every day along with other oils, I usually use 3-5 drops of OnGuard as a general preventive for infection and inflammation. Keeping infections at bay naturally and safely is reassuring and good for the body.

Toothpaste: I use the **Onguard** Toothpaste and it is amazingly cleansing for the mouth and it tastes great.

Counter, Hand and Laundry Cleanser: A few drops of **Onguard** oil in water in a spray bottle clean my counters and I put it in my detergent to clean and freshen laundry; I also use the foaming hand soap in the bathroom.

Frankincense is another oil I have come to appreciate and love. The herb Frankincense has been documented and used since 1500 BC by physicians and priests. It has been called LIQUID GOLD since it helps so many conditions from mood to acne and skin lesions and studies have shown it even has benefits for cancer. The gum resin is extracted from Boswellia trees in Oman for the doTERRA oils. Frankincense has been and still is a major trading commodity. In ancient days, tons of frankincense was transported by camels port to port because people valued it so highly for its amazing benefits.

General Wellbeing: I use 1-2 drops of **Frankincense** every morning on each of my feet after my bath and let the oils absorb in well through the larger pores. I also add 3-5 drops to my daily capsule of oil with **Onguard**.

Candida Suppression: I usually add 2-3 drops of **Oregano** to my oral capsule for suppressing yeast.

Drinking Water or Tea: I use 2-3 drops of **Lemon, Lime or Slim and Sassy** oil in my water or tea.

Facial Cleansing: I add 1 drop of **Lemon** into soapy hands before I scrub my face to dissolve oils and grime from the skin and pores. I usually add it to **Onguard** for cleaning sprays.

Sinus Congestion and Allergies: I inhale a few drops of **Peppermint** after rubbing them in my palms for alertness and opening up the sinuses for congestion or allergies.

Sleep and Relaxation: For sleep and calming at night I use **Lavender** on my feet, pillow and rub in palms and inhale.

Pet Use: I also use **Lavender** on the pads of my dog's feet for calming effect. **Sprains, Sore Muscles, and Headaches**: **Deep Blue** is an oil for topical use only and also comes as a cream. I have used it for sprained ankles, sore muscles and on the temples for headaches. It has fabulous properties for discomfort and inflammation.

For even more information, you can check out the extensive benefits and uses of OnGuard and Frankincense and any other oils of interest at www.everythingessential.me. You can also look up symptoms or conditions and see recommended oils.

If interested, ABC Wellness carries these oils at: www.mydoterra.com/abcwellness.

BONUS: PAW PAW EXTRACT – A SUPPLEMENT TO HELP YOU LIVE TO 100

Fabulous Nutrients from Nature's Sunshine: Have you heard about the Paw Paw? Strange name, yes, but it just might be a supplement you can use occasionally in your quest to live to the ripe old age of 100. Paw Paw tastes like a cross between a banana and a mango and Paw Paw trees grow in 26 states in the United States, growing wild from the Gulf Coast up to the Great Lakes region.

The Paw Paw fruit has yellow-green skin and soft, orange flesh which has earned it the nickname "custard apple," but it also goes by "poor man's banana" and "Indiana banana." This fruit has a creamy, custard-like consistency and a delicious, sweet flavor. Here is a picture, and you can google "Paw Paw" for more information.

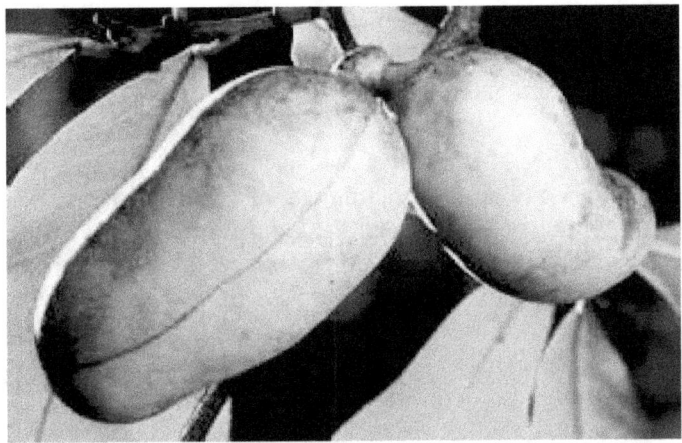

Paw Paw Cell-Reg by Nature's Sunshine: Now if you can find the fruit locally, you can enjoy it as a that way, but if not, you do have the option to take advantage of its benefits by taking capsules that contain an extract from the Paw Paw tree's twigs.

Benefits of Paw Paw:

1. Supports the immune system.
2. Selectively affects specific cells.
3. Modulates ATP production in specific cells.
5. Modulates blood supply to specific cells.

How Paw Paw Works:

The active compounds in Paw Paw Cell-Reg are a mixture of over 50 acetogenins. Acetogenins are active compounds that affect the production of ATP (Adenosine Triphosphate) in the mitochondria (the powerhouse) of the cell. ATP is the cells' major source of energy. Acetogenins selectively modulate the production of ATP in specific cells. Modulating the production of ATP affects the viability of specific cells and may help modulate the blood supply to them. Acetogenins also support and enhance the effectiveness of conventional medical regimens.

A clinical study with over 100 participants showed that the Paw Paw extract, containing a mixture of acetogenins, supports the body's normal cells during times of cellular stress. Paw Paw Cell-Reg is the only standardized acetogenin product available to regulate specific cells. Nature's Sunshine uses an extract of the twigs of the North American Paw Paw tree, which contain the most concentrated amount of acetogenins. These twigs are harvested when they are most biologically active, and the extract is standardized biologically using an invertebrate bioassay. This is a renewable resource since the tree is not harmed during the harvest.

Ingredients: Paw Paw twig extract.

Recommended Use: Take 2 capsules with food three times daily. Do not exceed recommended serving size or nausea may occur.

NOTE: Co-Q10, Thyroid Support and 7-Keto may decrease the effectiveness of this product. Only those with cellular abnormalities should take this product on a regular/daily basis. Do not take this product if you are pregnant, think you may become pregnant, or if you are breastfeeding.

How to Obtain Paw Paw Capsules: Go to www.naturessunshine.com Search Paw Paw. At check-out you can either pay retail or join the company and get the Wholesale price. If you prefer the wholesale discount, please join under Dr. Culik.

The ID to join under Dr. Culik is 3232529

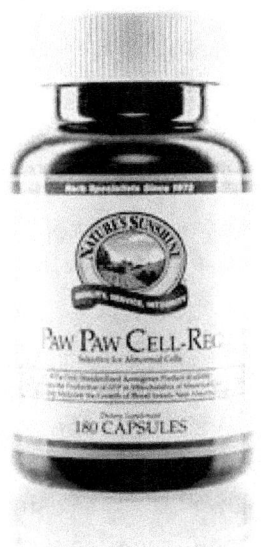

Bonus: Diet and Exercise

At this point, you want to focus on diet and exercise and you can follow your favorite program if you have one, but for those who don't I have supplied references for both diet and exercise, and you are free to investigate and follow any of these as I recommend them highly. We will also recommend another program at the end if you want more of a coaching program. Whatever plan you choose, I would suggest you follow just one plan at a time; using elements of other plans is OK though if the plan you are following provides no guidance.

Basic Nutritional Plan Recommended

After all the evaluations, we now move on to diet and exercise. First, we will start with a basic nutritional plan for you to follow unless you have received other guidance from a qualified expert:

1) Lots of purified water
2) Protein Breakfast within 1 hour of awakening
3) Protein at every meal
4) Protein shake at least 1/day per food sensitivities
5) Greens and Fruits Powders- for nutrients and alkalinity
6) Avoid Simple carbs: bread, rice, potatoes, pasta
7) No sugar even natural: Ok <u>B-Sweet</u> or Xylitol
8) Low glycemic veggies 3-6 per day

The beauty of the ABC Wellness Weightloss Pyramid method is it allows you to adopt any other methods you wish to try as far as diet and exercise – this plan is going to make all those other methods work better and faster because it is about eliminating problem areas that once held you back. But for those without a specific plan to follow, what comes next here is basic information gained from various experts and this should serve you well if you just want to follow this advice!

First, I just listed out a quick nutritional plan that includes lots of pure water, a protein breakfast within one hour of awakening, it may be a protein shake (have one shake per day), protein in every meal, greens or fruit powders, which are great for energy, avoiding the simple carbs like bread, rice, potatoes, pasta, and using either no sugar, or a healthy, safe sweetener like Boresha's B-Sweet or xylitol, and lots of low glycemic veggies 3-6 times per day.

DIET PLANS AVAILABLE

Here are some diet references for your convenience. These are healthy, low carb and Paleo type diets that can really make a difference for you!

1) **www.thepaleodiet.com** **Dr. Loren Cordain***
2) **www.jonnybowden.com** **Weight Loss Plans***
3) **www.theprimalblueprint.com** **web site and book**
4) **www.marksdailyapple.com** **free primal recipes**
5) **www.drhyman.com** **The Blood Sugar Solution Book and Cookbook**

6) **www.tanaamen.com** **The Omni Diet Book, wife of Dr. Daniel Amen Tana is an RN and fitness expert**
7) Also: We have a Registered Dietician and Weight Loss Expert Available at ABC Wellness...

See if any of these make sense for your particular situation. We recommend a low-carb diet, like a Paleo Diet, and there are several references here like Jonny Bowden, Primal Blue Print, and Dr. Hyman, who has a lot of information on sugar and the low glycemic diet, and there is a new book out called the Omni Diet by Dr. Tana's wife. For those interested and those in the local area, ABC Wellness has a dietitian here who does take individual patients and discusses nutrients and a diet specifically for them.

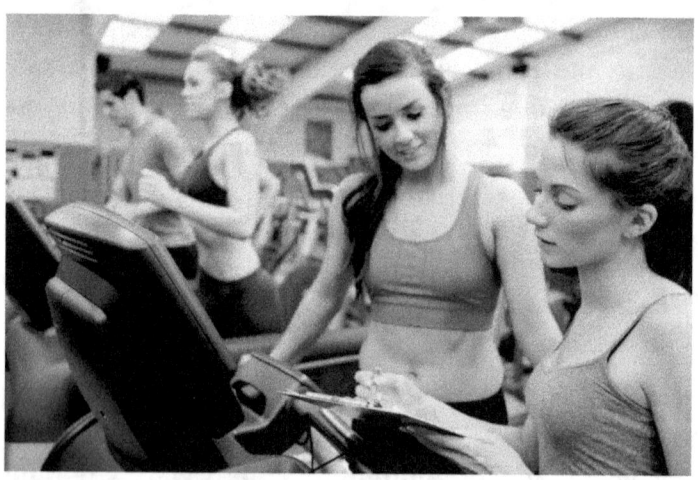

EXERCISE PLANS

1) Aerobic Exercise: Walk, Treadmill, Swim, Bike
2) Muscle building Anaerobic: Weights/Resistance
3) www.alsearsmd.com Dr. Al Sears PACE plan
4) Not monotonous cardio exercises but quick 10 minute routines with variable Pace.
5) Start a time, place, partner and put it on your schedule. At least 3 times a week and increase time and intensity.

About exercise plans, you are pretty much free to devise your own program, or use your favorite trainer's routine although we will make one recommendation to think about.

To start out, whether it is for five minutes or half an hour, just get yourself moving! You can begin with walking, using a treadmill, swimming, biking, or even doing some muscle building and weights, but start slow and easy and build up gradually whatever you decide to do. There is no use going overboard like some folks do when they first start a new routine. An injury to yourself will just set you back and is not worth it.

That said, you may want to consider the PACE plan as referenced. I love this book, and Dr. Al Sears is a doctor that recommends quick, maximum energy outputs, and to do short routines instead of the general walking or aerobics for five hours. He says you can get the energy and build it up fast and more naturally when you do like our ancestors did, kind of like the Paleo diet, but this is Paleo Exercise!

You know, our ancestors might chase that wild animal for 10 minutes, and then walk. And they probably weren't jogging for hours or days, just a short amount of time. So consider using this kind of routine – it might be easier to stick on this kind of routine long term, which is crucial for long term results and keeping the weight off.

Did You Like This Book?

Let everyone know by posting a review on Amazon. Just click here and it will take you to the review page; just scroll to the bottom.

SPECIAL ADDITION: BONUS ARTICLES!

To supplement the material above, we have included some articles pulled from our website at www.abcwellnessnews.com. We hope you find them informative and helpful. Some of the information is the same as what you learned, but more details have been added, and more explanation in terms of detail is given. Here is the list again as it appears in the table of contents at the beginning of this book:

Thyroid Adrenal Support – Iodine, Vitamin D – You are Probably Deficient!

Thyroid and Adrenal Glands – Gut Healing Nutrients, Vitamin C and Seasalt Supplements for Support

Thyroid Adrenal Support – Detoxification and Sleep as Health Aids!

THYROID ADRENAL DISEASE TESTING – 5 TIPS FOR PROPER DIAGNOSIS! PART 1 OF 2

March 11, 2013 Thyroid and Adrenal Care No Comments

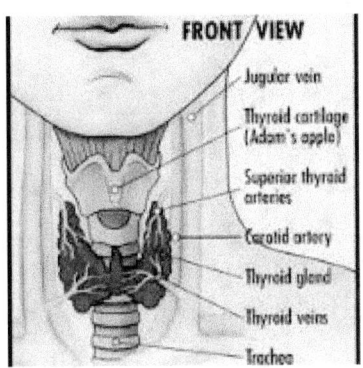

Has your thyroid and adrenal disease been missed or mistreated? There are an estimated 60,000,000+ people today with undiagnosed hypothyroidism. Discover what it takes to get properly tested.

Due to many factors, some beyond our control, we don't always recognize that we may have a problem with our thyroid or adrenal glands. And doctors often miss the diagnosis of hypothyroidism; testing really needs to be done in a specific way in order to determine if a low performing thyroid is affecting you.

Today we will talk about five different factors that are important in testing your thyroid – different things you need to know about and really think about to evaluate your thyroid properly. This will be part one of two articles on testing for thyroid.

1. Complete thyroid blood testing. A TSH is not adequate to decide if you have thyroid disease. You really must know not only your free T3, free T4, TSH, your thyroid antibodies, which include TPO and ATG, and you have to have reverse T3 to see if you have inactive thyroid production. Anyone of those may be enough to indicate that you have thyroid disease. So if you don't have the whole panel, your physician isn't doing enough to evaluate your thyroid.

2. Complete thyroid exam. Thyroid disease can be picked up on your blood work, but also many suggestions from your physical exam will suggest you have thyroid problems. You have to examine the skin for dryness, flakiness, itching, hair thinning, nails can be pitted, eyebrows, lateral brow thinning is a common problem, the thyroid gland itself can show

nodularity, enlargement, sometimes this is subtle, sometimes very severe. And pretibial edema or just some mild pitting or denting of the legs when you press on them with your thumb and also the reflexes of the lower extremities can affect the and be an indication of thyroid problems.

3. Thyroid questionnaire. This tool may be a significant help in indicating if you have thyroid problems, and will be provided after these first two articles on testing. So, you really need to go through this one by one, check off the ones that seem relevant to you, and take this to a thyroid, open minded physician, who can evaluate all your symptoms. So we have looked at your labs, your physical findings, and now your symptoms all by themselves may be a strong indicator.

4. Body temperature. Checking your basal body temperature is very important in evaluating if you have thyroid concerns, since the thyroid gland sets the metabolic rate. So to check you thyroid, you test in the morning for your temperature, letting you evaluate how your temperature is

compared to normal, which should be 98.6, or maybe minus a degree, but if it is less than 97.6, than you really have significance for possible thyroid issues. Many people run 96 or 95 and their doctors tell them, "that's just the way you are, your temperature runs low." But usually there is a reason for it and most often it's because your thyroid isn't completely functioning.

5. Food allergy testing. This is something critical if there is any concern with thyroid disease and especially if you have elevated thyroid antibodies, but food allergies are so common today that probably everyone should have them done. And this has to be blood work with IGG or IGA blood tests, the skin test or IGE blood tests that an allergist might do, or a pulmonary specialist are going to have nothing to do with whether your food allergies are significant related to your thyroid. Those are going to be related to peanut allergy or asthma problems. But you have to specifically ask for and get IG or IGA blood tests, especially for gluten, which is related to wheat, and casein, which is a protein in dairy.

That's it for today – 5 tips on proper testing for thyroid and adrenal disease. Please stay tuned for more testing tips in article number two to follow shortly.

Thank-you for your attention,

Diane Culik, MD
ABC Wellness

Diane A. Culik, MD, reveals secrets you really should know and promotes simple steps to greater health using natural, alternative methods. With Dr. Culik, you get the credibility and safety of a trained medical doctor, and the cutting edge alternative treatments of a Holistic Practitioner. For a free video on "Top 10 Things to Know about Thyroid and Adrenals before You Visit Your Doctor," please visit http://thyroid-adrenal-solutions.com. © Diane A. Culik, all rights reserved worldwide.

THYROID ADRENAL DISEASE TESTING – 6 MORE TIPS FOR PROPER DIAGNOSIS! PART 2 OF 2

March 12, 2013 Thyroid and Adrenal Care No Comments

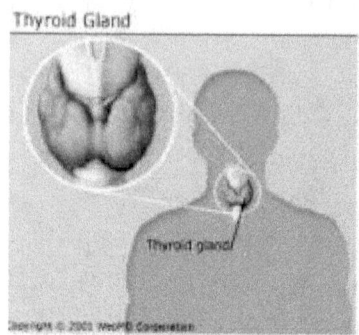

Has your thyroid and adrenal disease been missed or mistreated? There are an estimated 60,000,000+ people today with undiagnosed hypothyroidism. Discover what it takes to get properly tested; this is part 2 of 2 articles on thyroid adrenal disease testing.

In this second article, we continue with 6 more critical or major tests you should address if you really want to know what is going on with your thyroid and adrenal glands. While there is other thyroid adrenal disease testing that could be helpful, having these tests done should be a great start on assessing status and determining what kind of actions you can take to improve the functioning of your thyroid and adrenal glands.

Your overall health will also be much improved if you can address any factors where you have subpar thyroid or adrenal performance occurring, as these glands affect the entire body.

1. Basic Food Allergy Testing. If you have any food allergy findings, anything positive, you really should see a nutritionist, and especially a holistic nutritionist to help you review what you are eating, what you can change, and how you can revise your diet. If there are several food allergies that are elevated, you may want to consider a complete blood panel of IGG blood testing, and several of the laboratories like Bio Tek are able to do that from even just a little finger stick of blood.

2. Heavy Metal Testing. This should definitely be done if you have any amalgams or silver fillings, if you eat or every ate any significant amount of fish, certainly if you have exposures, just being near a coal factory that is coal burning, and certainly if you have any neurological symptoms, any tremor, any symptoms of Parkinson's, multiple

sclerosis, any brain fog, chronic fatigue, fibromyalgia, as all of these can be related to heavy metal toxicity.

3. Vitamin Testing. This is very essential, and the things that are most related to thyroid problems are zinc levels, and especially RBC, red blood cells zinc level is important, you serum selenium is significant, those are both required for thyroid conversion in the cells to the active form (T4 to T3 conversion). And B vitamins are also essential, it is especially easy to measure B1, B6, and B12.

4. Comprehensive Analysis of Intracellular Nutrients. For more complete testing, there are labs such as Spectra-Cell that can do a very comprehensive analysis of intracellular nutrients, and they will measure 33 different vitamins, many that you can't get from a regular lab such as vitamin C, vitamin K, vitamin E, certainly all the B vitamins, but also Biotin, CoQ10, Alpha-Lipoic Acid, selenium, chromium, calcium, which is the only way to get an accurate level, not possible from traditional labs, magnesium, zinc, copper, glutathione, Carnitine, serine, glutamine, on and on. So this is a very helpful test, and everyone I have tested so far has one,

and usually several, deficiencies that are essential for maximizing your health.

5. Saliva Testing for Adrenals. If you have concerns and you're not sure, there are several companies including Diagnostics that will do a saliva test – a little spit 4 times during the day, and they can even measure your DHEA and cortisol as it fluctuates through the daytime and evening, and this is really much more accurate than one single blood test at one point in time. And it will tell you if you are having adrenal fatigue or adrenal burnout, or high cortisol, maybe high stress, both of these may be detrimental to your thyroid function.

6. Complete Panel for Food Allergies. Again for food allergies, if you have one or two of the common food allergens such as gluten or casein you may want to consider a whole panel, because often with leaky gut there may be other foods that have caused problems and you have become allergic to them. Several companies, including Bio-Tek will do 96 different food allergens by IGG from just several drops of blood and you can even do this test at home – just a finger stick and put a drop of blood on a little card, dry it

and send it off. So it is a fabulous way to get a very complete analysis, with minimal cost and time.

In summary, these tests, combined with the first five will provide a comprehensive picture of your thyroid and adrenal health. By knowing in depth what is going on, you can then move on to specific action steps to address any deficiencies, and work to correct any imbalances.

In the next article, we will provide a checklist questionnaire that will allow you to determine for yourself if you may have thyroid and adrenal concerns. If you score positively on many factors listed on the questionnaire, then it may be worth pursuing the additional testing that we wrote about in this article and the last one.

Thank-you for reading,

Diane Culik, MD
ABC Wellness

Diane A. Culik, MD, reveals secrets you really should know and promotes simple steps to greater health using natural, alternative methods. With Dr. Culik, you get the credibility and safety of a trained medical doctor, and the cutting edge alternative treatments of a Holistic Practitioner. For a free video on "Top 10 Things to Know about Thyroid and Adrenals before You Visit Your Doctor," please visit http://thyroid-adrenal-solutions.com. © Diane A. Culik, all rights reserved worldwide.

HYPOTHYROIDISM QUESTIONNAIRE – IS THYROID ADRENAL DISEASE A CONCERN FOR YOU?

March 13, 2013 Thyroid and Adrenal Care No Comments

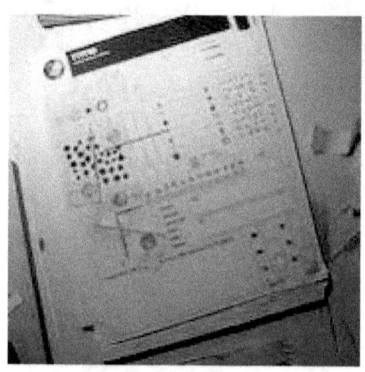

Has your thyroid and adrenal disease been missed or mistreated? There are an estimated 60,000,000+ people today with undiagnosed hypothyroidism. Use this hypothyroidism questionnaire to determine if your thyroid and/or adrenal glands are underperforming.

In the last 2 articles, we covered 11 major thyroid and adrenal disease testing methods that would let you ascertain if you have thyroid or adrenal issues. Some of these tests would give you helpful information concerning the status of your overall health regardless of whether it was thyroid or adrenal in nature. So there would be some value in doing these tests regardless.

However, before deciding if you even need to conduct such tests, you can first use this thyroid and adrenal questionnaire to determine if you actually do have thyroid problems or adrenal problems, and if pursuing the thyroid tests listed in the last 2 articles is warranted. Here is the thyroid adrenal questionnaire – please print this out, and place a checkmark by each positive response.

Hypothyroidism Questionnaire and Symptom Evaluation (check any positives)

(_____) Sensitivity to cold or hands and feet are usually cold

(_____) Morning temperatures are less than 97.8

(_____) Wear socks to bed often

(_____) Dry or scaly skin

(_____) Need to apply lotion and oils frequently

(_____) Often daily fatigue

(_____) Never seem to get enough sleep or naps for energy

(_____) Memory and concentration are decreased

(_____) Hair is thinning, course, dry, breaking off

(_____) Nails are thin, chip, peal or break

(_____) Lower legs are puffy, or indent with pressure

(_____) Hands and fingers are puffy

(_____) Carpel Tunnel symptoms

(_____) Outer third of eyebrows are thin or absent

(_____) Libido or sex drive has decreased or is low

(_____) Weight is difficult to lose or gain even when dieting

(_____) Bowels are sluggish or constipated or need to take laxatives

(_____) Autoimmune diseases like Rheumatoid, Lupus, and Vitiligo

(_____) Low B12 or Pernicious Anemia

(_____) Known or suspected food allergies or Celiac Disease

(_____) Silver Amalgams now or in the past (mercury fillings)

(_____) History of radiation therapy to neck or chest

(_____) Drinking now or prior, water with chlorine and/or fluoride

(_____) Eat moderate amounts of soy milk, cheese, burgers, dressings, etc.

(_____) Family History of any type of Thyroid Problems

(_____) Eat fish frequently esp. tuna, sushi, non-wild Salmon

(_____) Moody, depressed, irritable, apathetic

(_____) Fatigue on waking even after good night's sleep

(_____) Use of Teflon Pans

(_____) Using white salt instead of gray or pink unprocessed salt

(_____) Craving caffeine as soon as you awaken…or hard to get started

(_____) Second wind in evening and may be up late and hard to sleep

(_____) Leg cramps and charley horse symptoms

(_____) Puffy eyelids

(_____) Sluggish bowels…may need laxatives and softeners

(_____) Use Mountain Dew or Bromo Seltzer

(_____) Use hot tubs with chlorine or bromine

(_____) May struggle to push through several hours of activity after waking

How did you do? Less than 3 or 4, you are probably fine in the thyroid adrenal area, but if you scored positive on 5 to 9, you probably have some moderate thyroid issues. If you scored 10 or higher, your thyroid and adrenals could definitely use some attention. The prevalence of things that are toxic to your thyroid and adrenal glands and the nutritional deficiencies in most people's diets is overwhelming – hence the huge number of undiagnosed persons walking around with hypothyroidism that could help themselves feel much better through prudent action.

One tip is to immediately cut back on anything bad for your thyroid like soy or excessive fish, and see if you feel better in a week or two. Another is to add a tablespoon or two of coconut oil, which is good for your thyroid, to your daily routine.

Stay tuned, as we will cover things to avoid and things that enhance thyroid and adrenal health in upcoming articles – you will not want to miss these super alternative, natural health tips!

Thank-you for joining us,

Diane Culik, MD
ABC Wellness

Diane A. Culik, MD, reveals secrets you really should know and promotes simple steps to greater health using natural, alternative methods. With Dr. Culik, you get the credibility and safety of a trained medical doctor, and the cutting edge alternative treatments of a Holistic Practitioner. For a free video on "Top 10 Things to Know about Thyroid and Adrenals before You Visit Your Doctor," please visit http://thyroid-adrenal-solutions.com. © Diane A. Culik, all rights reserved worldwide.

THYROID ADRENAL HEALTH – 7 TOXIC THINGS TO AVOID! PART 1 OF 3

March 14, 2013 Thyroid and Adrenal Care No Comments

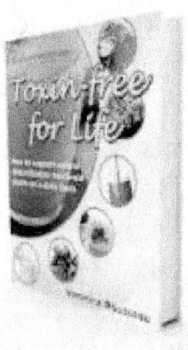

Has your thyroid and adrenal disease been missed or mistreated? There are an estimated 60,000,000+ people today with undiagnosed hypothyroidism. Discover which toxic things may be affecting your thyroid and adrenal health. This is part 1 of 3 articles.

As with all things, don't go overboard with all these suggestions. It would drive you crazy trying to eliminate every one of these items out of your life. However, you can probably work on identifying and reducing the major toxic offenders in your situation. Doing so will guarantee a positive result in your health. Why? Because when the toxic burden is lessened, the thyroid, adrenals, and all other organs have to work less hard to maintain a healthy state. It is when the body is overloaded with toxins that a state of disease results.

Here is a list of things that have or may have a negative effect on our thyroid and adrenals glands. Although there may be toxic items that are not shown here, please check out this list and see if there are any items you can take action on. Also examine your life for other toxins not on this list that can be reduced or eliminated.

Thyroid and Adrenal Health – Toxic Things to Avoid

1. Soy. Of course, you know about Soy Milk and Soy Beans, but Soy is also hidden in many foods, such as dressings and processed foods.
2. Fluoride. You are probably going to have this in your tap water, your shower, fluoride added toothpaste and mouthwash, so you want to get natural sources and filter your water.
3. Bromine. Unfortunately, for as much as it is used in our foods, bromine is very toxic. Bromo-Seltzer, brominated hot tubs, pretty much any processed flour now has bromine in it.

4. Chlorine. We find this in our tap water, and though it is great to kill off bacteria, it damages the good bacteria in our gut and interferes with iodine.

5. PFOAs and Teflon. Teflon and PFOAs are also toxic and interfere with our thyroid. These are usually going to be in either plastic bottles or coated pans.

6. Mercury amalgams. Silver fillings have 50% mercury in them, and mercury is not good for your thyroid; it also interferes with the T4 to T3 conversion process.

7. Flu shots and vaccines. These often had mercury in them also in the form of thimerosol, and even though many vaccines have taken them out, there is still mercury in some vaccines they give adults as well as pregnant women and children..

And that's it to start – 7 things that may be serving as toxins to your thyroid and adrenal glands; items you can work on reducing or eliminating from your life to see if you feel better, or if you feel good, to feel fantastic. In any case, taking these steps now will keep you healthier and stronger for a much longer time, letting you live life to its fullest.

Please stay with us as the next couple articles will identify more toxins that affect the functioning of your thyroid and adrenal glands.

Thank-you for your attention,

Diane Culik, MD
ABC Wellness

Diane A. Culik, MD, reveals secrets you really should know and promotes simple steps to greater health using natural, alternative methods. With Dr. Culik, you get the credibility and safety of a trained medical doctor, and the cutting edge alternative treatments of a Holistic Practitioner. For a free video on "Top 10 Things to Know about Thyroid and Adrenals before You Visit Your Doctor," please visit http://thyroid-adrenal-solutions.com. © Diane A. Culik, all rights reserved worldwide.

THYROID ADRENAL HEALTH – 7 MORE TOXIC THINGS TO AVOID! PART 2 OF 3

March 19, 2013 Thyroid and Adrenal Care No Comments

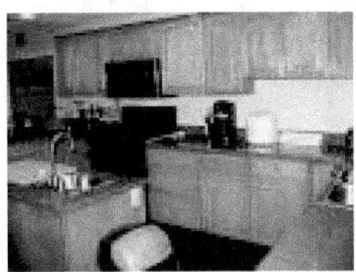

Has your thyroid and adrenal disease been missed or mistreated? There are an estimated 60,000,000+ people today with undiagnosed hypothyroidism. Discover which toxic things may be affecting your thyroid and adrenal health. This is part 2 of 3 articles.

This article continues with more possibilities as to what may be affecting your health in a negative manner. It is not always easy to discern whether your thyroid and adrenals are an issue for you, but it is helpful to know that adequate thyroid hormone is being produced and available in the blood.

First of all, why should you care about thyroid hormone levels in the blood? Because thyroid hormone must be present in adequate amounts to feel good. Toxins interfere with production of thyroid hormone, and because thyroid hormone affects virtually every cell in the body, having too little of this hormone in the blood can slow the body down. This is called hypothyroidism, and symptoms are numerous with major hypothyroid symptoms showing as weight gain, fatigue, depression and hair loss, as well as many other problems.

To continue, let's give you just a bit more information in case your doctor or someone else speaks to you about hypothyroidism. The purpose of the thyroid gland is to make, store, and release thyroid hormone into your blood. This hormone affects nearly all your cells and if too little exists in the blood you are hypothyroid. Too much thyroid hormone is called hyperthyroidism. We will reveal more facts on thyroid in the next article.

So for today, here it is – list number two with 7 more things that have or may have a negative effect on our thyroid and adrenal glands. Also, please remember to examine your life for other toxins not on this list that can be reduced or eliminated.

Thyroid and Adrenal Health – 7 More Toxic Things to Avoid

1. Fish. Basically limit your intake to Wild Pacific Salmon; all other fish are going to have mercury in them and not worth the risk. If you do eat other seafood, at least try to keep it as an occasional thing.

2. Cabbage. Try to limit foods that use any plants in the cabbage family. These contain chemicals called pro-goitrins which may affect thyroid function.

3. Processed Foods. As you know, eat as close to nature as possible, and avoid refined, manmade foods. Most food additives that extend shelf life are not good for you.

4. Deodorants. Most of these contain toxic elements such as aluminum, so check the ingredient list, and choose one that is natural. There are coconut based products available.

5. Hair Dye. Again, find a natural one if you can.

6. Sugar and sugar substitutes. Aspartame and other sweeteners can be toxic. Perhaps try stevia, which is a natural sweetener.

7. Negative emotions and stress. It has been proven that our minds affect our bodies, so work on staying stress free. Eliminate clutter from your life if you can.

And that's it – 7 more things that may be serving as toxins to your thyroid and adrenal glands. Please stay with us for the last article which presents another 7 toxins that affect the functioning of your thyroid and adrenals.

Thank-you for reading,

Diane Culik, MD
ABC Wellness

Diane A. Culik, MD, reveals secrets you really should know and promotes simple steps to greater health using natural, alternative methods. With Dr. Culik, you get the credibility and safety of a trained medical doctor, and the cutting edge alternative treatments of a Holistic Practitioner. For a free video on "Top 10 Things to Know about Thyroid and Adrenals before You Visit Your Doctor," please visit http://thyroid-adrenal-solutions.com. © Diane A. Culik, all rights reserved worldwide.

THYROID ADRENAL HEALTH – FINAL TOXIC THINGS TO AVOID! PART 3 OF 3

March 20, 2013 Thyroid and Adrenal Care No Comments

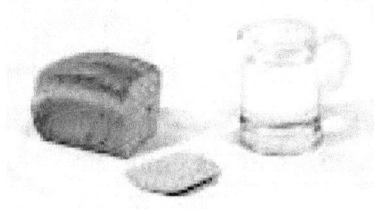

Has your thyroid and adrenal disease been missed or mistreated? There are an estimated 60,000,000+ people today with undiagnosed hypothyroidism. Discover the truth about more toxic things that may negatively affect thyroid and adrenal function. This is part 3 of 3 articles.

In this final article, we present an additional 7 items that can be toxic to your thyroid and adrenals. We have tried to present the major or critical offenders in each article presented, and although there is some overlap in what we have written, we hope you have gained some valuable insight into what may be affecting your thyroid and/or adrenal health.

Once again, the purpose of the thyroid gland is to make, store and release thyroid hormone into your blood. But let's talk about some related glands. The amount of thyroid hormone made by your pituitary, as well as part of your brain called the hypothalamus, adjusts the amount of thyroid hormone made by your thyroid gland. The pituitary, aided by the hypothalamus, controls many of your glands, as well as helping to control other bodily functions such as thirst, hunger, sleep and body temperature.

All three of these glands need to work together to control the amount of thyroid hormone in your body at any given time. When toxins get into any of these glands or any of our body's critical areas they may affect the production of hormones and other things our bodies need to function properly. Our purpose here is not to overwhelm you with information, but just to give you some basic data that you can put to use in your daily life. It's by knowing what toxins might be affecting you that you can take action and hopefully gain a positive result.

Here is the final list for now of things that have or may have a negative effect on our thyroid and adrenal glands.

Thyroid and Adrenal Health – Some Final Toxic Things to Avoid

1. Smoking. You know how toxic this can be to your health, and especially the thyroid.
2. Radiation. In any form, it affects the thyroid and adrenals negatively.
3. Wheat. Processed wheat breads contain gluten as a major ingredient, which causes inflammation, and stresses the thyroid.
4. Environmental Toxins. Try to avoid exposure to pesticides and other toxic chemicals used around the house and yard.
5. Over medication – Avoid prescription medicines whenever possible – they often cause worse side effects than the issues they treat.
6. Starvation or overeating carbohydrates. Radical diet changes may affect thyroid function, adrenal function too.
7. Vegetarianism – small amounts of animal protein help the thyroid and adrenals function. If you do go vegetarian, consider supplementing with proteins, extra coconut oil, and other items.

There you have it − 7 additional things that may be serving as unwanted burdens in your life, and may need to be addressed as to reducing or eliminating exposure. This finishes our discourse for now on toxins that affect the functioning of your thyroid and adrenal glands. Future articles are planned on supplements and ways to support your thyroid and adrenals, so please stay tuned.

Thank-you again for your interest,

Diane Culik, MD
ABC Wellness

Diane A. Culik, MD, reveals secrets you really should know and promotes simple steps to greater health using natural, alternative methods. With Dr. Culik, you get the credibility and safety of a trained medical doctor, and the cutting edge alternative treatments of a Holistic Practitioner. For a free video on "Top 10 Things to Know about Thyroid and Adrenals before You Visit Your Doctor," please visit http://thyroid-adrenal-solutions.com. © Diane A. Culik, all rights reserved worldwide.

THYROID ADRENAL SUPPORT – IODINE, VITAMIN D – YOU ARE PROBABLY DEFICIENT!

March 25, 2013 Thyroid and Adrenal Care No Comments

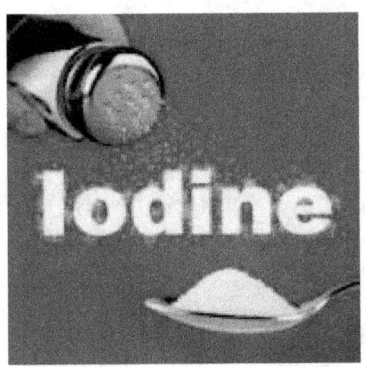

Has your thyroid and adrenal disease been missed or mistreated? There are an estimated 60,000,000+ people today with undiagnosed hypothyroidism. Discover how Iodine and Vitamin D really help the thyroid and adrenal glands function at optimal levels.

We start with two vital elements needed for thyroid and adrenal support – Iodine and Vitamin D. Number one, your body does not make Iodine, and your thyroid absolutely needs Iodine, which is supplied through diet, to function properly. Number two, also for thyroid, Vitamin D plays an important support role. Now let me make what is perhaps a disturbing statement, "You are most probably deficient in Iodine and maybe Vitamin D too!"

Yes, it may be true – studies conducted in Michigan showed over 95% of those tested had low Iodine levels, and Iodine is critical for proper thyroid functioning. Some say this is a global problem, and it may be a shame, because Iodine is available and cheap. If so many Michigan residents are deficient, we can assume those in nearby areas are too. After all, this was part of what was known as the "Goiter Belt" years ago, where persons would show up at their doctor's with enlarged necks due to their thyroid not receiving enough iodine. The Iodine had been depleted out of the soil. That's why Iodine or Iodide was originally added to our salt.

Perhaps you live elsewhere, but it is likely that by today most soils lack Iodine and other critical nutrients like Selenium, which aids the thyroid as well. So Iodine is critical for everybody, but absolutely essential if you have thyroid problems. Our bodies don't get enough from the salt that we eat. We have currently added Iodine to the diet through salt enhancement, but the problem is it is only added in small amounts to the white salt we consume. Unfortunately, this white salt has been processed and all the minerals have been removed.

So what you want to do is use only the unprocessed, natural sea salt that is usually pink or gray. This will have no Iodine, so to raise your levels, what you really need to do is mimic what the Japanese people do, and take Iodine pills or eat sea vegetables, or take kelp tablets and try to get your Iodine intake up to 10,000 or 12,000 mg per day, which is the average for the Japanese, who live longer on this planet than any other nationality. They also have the lowest rate of breast cancer in any developed nation for their women.

Iodine is what your thyroid uses to create thyroid hormones, either 3 or 4 Iodine molecules, and all the other chemicals we are exposed to like bromine, fluoride, and chlorine interfere and block this Iodine we are getting, so we need to make sure we are getting adequate amounts to begin with to keep the thyroid functioning well.

Vitamin D is also very important for health, and many people show low levels when tested. Vitamin D helps your thyroid, it lowers breast cancer risk, and probably most cancer risks; it helps improve your immune system for flu, for infections, and it lowers the risk of diabetes, high blood pressure, and even multiple sclerosis. So your vitamin D Levels should be, that is, your 25 hydroxy Vitamin D levels should be, 50 to 80, and this is referenced per Dr. Hollick, who is a Vitamin D expert.

Studies have shown that women have 50% less breast cancer when their vitamin D level is 52 or above. So it's very important to work with your thyroid and your immune system by keeping your Vitamin D levels adequate too. Sunshine helps the body make Vitamin D, so if you live in areas where the sun is not available for long periods you may be deficient unless your dietary intake is high.

One tip is to get out in the sunshine for short periods daily – it really does help you feel better and be healthier. Just don't overdo it – you do not need hours a day in the sun, 20 or 30 minutes may be sufficient.

Thank-you for reading,

Diane Culik, MD
ABC Wellness

Diane A. Culik, MD, reveals secrets you really should know and promotes simple steps to greater health using natural, alternative methods. With Dr. Culik, you get the credibility and safety of a trained medical doctor, and the cutting edge alternative treatments of a Holistic Practitioner. For a free video on "Top 10 Things to Know about Thyroid and Adrenals before You Visit Your Doctor," please visit http://thyroid-adrenal-solutions.com. © Diane A. Culik, all rights reserved worldwide.

THYROID AND ADRENAL GLANDS – GUT HEALING NUTRIENTS, VITAMIN C AND SEASALT SUPPLEMENTS FOR SUPPORT

April 1, 2013 Thyroid and Adrenal Care No Comments

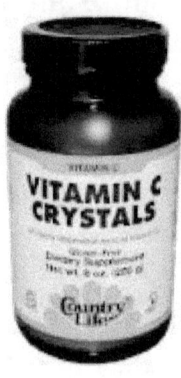

Has your thyroid and adrenal disease been missed or mistreated? There are an estimated 60,000,000+ people today with undiagnosed hypothyroidism. Discover how gut healing nutrients, vitamin C and sea salt really help the thyroid and adrenal glands do the job they were meant to do.

Here are 3 major ways to support your thyroid and adrenal glands. Taking these kinds of supplements will help you feel better in a number of ways, and your overall health will also be much improved if you can address any factors where you have subpar thyroid or adrenal performance occurring, as these glands affect the entire body.

1. Gut Healing Nutrients. There are several nutrients that are very important for gut healing, for healing inflammation, certainly if you have food allergies, if you have yeast, or if you have leaky gut and these items may include glutamine, the omega 3s, or Krill Oil. Aloe is very helpful, MSM, licorice can very helpful, and colostrum.

   Next, coconut oil is good for gut health, good for thyroid, good for improving your weight, and may even have some benefits for brain health. So coconut oil is another simple, easy thing that you can add as a nutrient into your body.

   Probiotics are essential probably for everyone, but certainly if there is gut inflammation, if you have food allergies, if you have yeast. Again, probiotics mean you are putting the good bacteria back in to replace the bad bacteria and yeast, and the function of the intestines is dramatically improved and probiotics even help for weight loss and for mood problems and mental health. So replace those bad bacteria with good bacteria by taking probiotics.

2. Vitamin C's Remarkable Properties. Vitamin C is good for every human being on the planet, and it's really critical for fatigue and especially for adrenal fatigue and adrenal burnout. Vitamin C is not made by human beings or other primates, and also fruit bats and guinea pigs are not able to make vitamin C in their liver, we lost the ability, so we need to take in more vitamin C than just to prevent scurvy and dying within a few months. We need it for our vascular system, our joints, our connective tissue, and absolutely for our adrenals – at least 2000 mg a day, is the preferred dose.

It is available from Life Extension, from Pure Encapsulations, and you can get it in capsules, sometimes powdered, buffered form, and even chewables. It's excellent for kids to adults, any age. For adults at least 2000 mg, children, 1000 mg would be reasonable.

3. Let's Talk Salt. Next, tip number three, salt is very important for the body. Our bodies require salt, and you need to use

> unprocessed sea salt that is not white, that has all the good trace minerals in it. It may be Celtic or Himalayan Salt from deep deposits in the earth that have all the preserved natural minerals.
>
> If you have white salt, it is not the right salt; it has been made to look good, but all the minerals have been removed. Sources (of unprocessed sea salt) are available from health food stores.

There you have it - 3 more super tips to put to use; these three supplements will provide a boost to your thyroid, adrenal, and perhaps overall health. As far as these and other supplements go, you may want to consider testing to see if you are deficient in any areas, thereby knowing what you need to be taking and what kind of dosage is appropriate. It is safe to say that most people would benefit from Vitamin C, coconut oil, omega 3s or Krill Oil, sea salt and probiotics at some level to start. Please catch our next article on Detoxification and Sleep where we will inform and educate on more ways to support thyroid and adrenal health.

Thank-you,

Diane Culik, MD
ABC Wellness

Diane A. Culik, MD, reveals secrets you really should know and promotes simple steps to greater health using natural, alternative methods. With Dr. Culik, you get the credibility and safety of a trained medical doctor, and the cutting edge alternative treatments of a Holistic Practitioner. For a free video on "Top 10 Things to Know about Thyroid and Adrenals before You Visit Your Doctor," please visit http://thyroid-adrenal-solutions.com. © Diane A. Culik, all rights reserved worldwide.

THYROID ADRENAL SUPPORT – DETOXIFICATION AND SLEEP AS HEALTH AIDS!

April 2, 2013 Thyroid and Adrenal Care No Comments

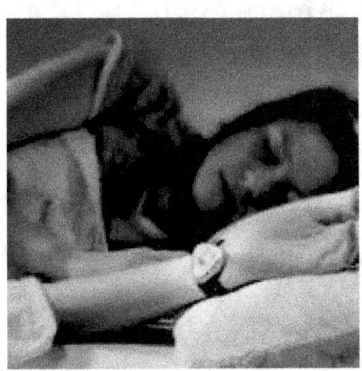

Hypothyroidism affects millions of people today without them even knowing it! Discover how detoxification and sleep really help the thyroid and adrenal glands recover from daily stress and let you feel your best.

Here are 2 more major ways to support your thyroid and adrenal glands. Taking these actions will help you feel better in a number of ways, and your overall health will also be much improved if you can address any factors where you have subpar thyroid or adrenal performance occurring, as these glands affect the entire body.

129

1. Detoxification Does a Body Good. Cleansing helps support the liver, the thyroid, the adrenals, and the rest of the body. You can detoxify with nutrients, such as Chlorella, and Cilantro, or you can do it with many different herbs including milk thistle, and other nutrients such as Alpha-Lipoic Acid. There are many other herbs and nutrients that are very helpful, so you may want to research anything you choose to use.

The suggestion is made to start with a trial first to see how you respond. There is a caveat with some nutrients such as chlorella and cilantro. Some practitioners believe these substances can stir mercury up and cause it to redistribute in the tissues, so proceed cautiously whenever using such items. Do this especially if you have a number of silver (mercury) amalgam fillings. It is recommended you have any silver fillings removed safely by a holistic dentist trained in proper removal, and replaced with safe materials. Ask your dentist to see the material safety data sheet for the filling material, and Google the ingredients for safety reasons.

Finally, whatever you finally choose to detox with, start with a very low dosage every few hours on a regular schedule and see how you do. There are support groups on the internet who will coach you in proper detoxification. Dr. Andy Cutler, a research scientist has written an excellent book on detoxing mercury from the body if you care to Google him as a resource – some consider him to be a premier authority on such issues. Detoxification products are available from Life Extension, and Pure Encapsulations.

2. Sleep Serves as a Super Health Aid. The final tip for today is that you really need adequate sleep to support your thyroid and adrenals, as well as your whole body. A recent study reported that 76% of Americans suffer with sleep problems, so please take note – catching up on your sleep is one of the quickest routes to feeling good again! So take some extra time to invest in yourself, and find some helpful supplements.

One great product is melatonin, you can start at 3 mg and you can double and triple the dose; it's very safe, and people with immune deficiencies or cancer can even take 20 or 40 mg daily. Other options include herbal teas, chamomile, valerian, hops, and GABA. GABA can be obtained in capsules, or now we even have the chewable GABA that not only helps with sleep, but with anxiety and stress disorders also.

OK, that's enough for today - 2 more super health tips to get started with; applying these tips will provide a boost to your thyroid, adrenal, and perhaps overall health. But please don't stop after a short trial – adequate sleep and regular cleansing of your body should be a way of life. Please catch our next article, where we will inform and educate on more super supplements for thyroid and adrenal health.

Thank-you for joining us,

Diane Culik, MD
ABC Wellness

Diane A. Culik, MD, reveals secrets you really should know and promotes simple steps to greater health using natural, alternative methods. With Dr. Culik, you get the credibility and safety of a trained medical doctor, and the cutting edge alternative treatments of a Holistic Practitioner. For a free video on "Top 10 Things to Know about Thyroid and Adrenals before You Visit Your Doctor," please visit http://thyroid-adrenal-solutions.com. © Diane A. Culik, all rights reserved worldwide.

Did You Like This Book?

Let everyone know by posting a review on Amazon. Just click here and it will take you to the reviews page; just scroll to the bottom.